Mystery, Magic And Medicine

How Emotional Trauma Results in Physical Disease and How to Reverse It

William W. Easley, D.C., D.Ch

Copyright © 2018 William W. Easley

All rights reserved. No part of this publication may be reproduced or transmitted in any form or by any means, electronic or mechanical, including photocopy, without written permission from the author. Reviewers may quote brief passages.

Cover art by: Navin Boopathi
colourkraft@gmail.com

First Printing Edition 2018

ISBN: 1719485720

ISBN-13: 978-1719485722

DEDICATION

To the advancement of the healing arts.

CONTENTS

Acknowledgements	9
Introduction	11
Food For Thought	17
Part One	
What are Health and Disease	19
How Disease Progresses	22
What are Therapeutics	24
Easley Energy Therapy	27
Classifications of disease	30
Differentiating between 2 levels of disease	33
Treatment of physically based disease	38
Treatment of energy based disease	40
The Overlap Factor	43
Part Two	
The Person as an Organism	49
The Structure of the Organism	53
The Importance of Symptoms	62
Treatment of Symptoms	64
How Physical Healing Works	67
Results of Types of Treatment	68
Energy-based and Physically-based Diseases	74
Part Three	
The Person as a Being	83
Structure of the Physical (Anatomy)	93
How the Being Works	96

The Importance of Symptoms	99
Treatment of Symptoms	102
How Energetic Disease Works	103
How Emotions are Involved in Health	108
How Energy Healing Works	117
Factors Involved in Physically Based Disease	122
How Your Lifestyle Affects Your Person	124
Factors Involved in Energy-based Disease	127
Part Four	
Relationships of the Energy Body to the Physical	137
Comparative Overview of Physical & Energy Systems	139
Which Part of the Person is in Charge	143
Why the Physical Conforms to the Subtle	144
How the Subtle Body Becomes Diseased	146
Part Five	
The Five Chinese Elements	149
Prana, Chi, Qi, The Great Spirit, and the Holy Spirit	151
Yin/Yang and The Five Elements	154
How The Elements Create Balance and Imbalance	157
The Result of the Imbalance of the Elements	160
Primary Pathological Emotions	162
Part Six	
The Challenge System of Discovery	165
Needed To Do This Adequately	169
Use of the Hands and the Mind	171
How to Assess a Meridian	174
Tonifying and Sedating	179

How Much is Enough? Too much?	182
When Not to Start	185
How Long Will a Treatment Last?	188
When a Problem Returns or Worsens	190
Part Seven	
How to Manage Very Complicated Cases	193
Pranic Healing, Pranic Psychotherapy, and Crystals	197
RyodoRaku: The Great Unraveller	203
Auriculotherapy	205
Classic Acupuncture	209
In Conclusion	210
Appendix	211
Explanation of Terms	219
Referenced Materials and Reading List	229

ACKNOWLEDGMENTS

To my Teachers, Grand Master Choa Kok Sui, Mahaguruji Mei Ling, the numerous masters of their respective arts, Dr. George Goodheart and Dr. Larry Jaggers in particular, my many professional colleagues and patients from whom I learned the true meaning of the word "practice" and so much more, and to all of those who have endured so much suffering in their lives due to the unhealthy state of our health care professions and society.

Much gratitude also to Anna Rhodes for her extensive help in editing the manuscript, and to Krista Terry for the final formatting and polishing.

Also, to my children, without them, my life would have been left without so much meaning.

INTRODUCTION

"Doctor, can you help me? I've been to four other specialists before I came to you, and I'm getting worse. No one has been able to help me." Does this sound familiar to you? Or possibly this, you have an "incurable" condition. Then the doctor says "You needn't worry too much about it though, we do have treatment. You will have to take this medication for the rest of your life, later on have a surgery due the unavoidable complications that will occur later, and your life span will not be shortened by too much, and maybe an amputation or two, or possibly numerous laser surgeries (as in the case of diabetes)."

Maybe you will live the rest of your life with your lifestyle severely altered by the effects of the drugs used to reduce your awareness of the pain (as with fibromyalgia). What about those with carpal tunnel syndrome, asthma, Crohn's disease, irritable bowel syndrome?

Consult with another physician and you are likely to hear "Well, we are still working on that one...and making great progress too. They think they have found either a virus or a gene that causes that problem." Right! Are you kidding me? They have been working on these things for decades on end and are no closer to a cure than they were 40 years ago, but treatments abound.

Then there's the "I'm going to refer you to another specialist. I think they might be able to help." Yes, they might. Usually, they help your medical bill go up another quantum level. Remember who is making the profit on this deal. Oh, I almost forgot to mention all of those expensive tests that they run. Interesting how the next doctor has to run them all over again. What was wrong with the first three rounds of tests? Usually nothing, but it really helps to spread the diagnostic money around (insurance companies quibble less about diagnostics than most of the other charges.)

If this sounds familiar to you or someone you know or you have been subjected to this type of care, please do three things for yourself.

First, take heart, there is hope! You may be able to take care of the problem yourself, or have another person help you out by utilizing a painless and effective method that can be learned by almost anyone of average intelligence.

Second, forgive the doctors previously seen. They are sincere professionals doing the best they know how and were just doing their job as they were trained. Their job is stressful, risky, often frustrating and they have to toe an unwritten line of which most people aren't aware.

Their job is usually not fun. Let's face the fact that they work in the unforgiving realm of a mixture of physically-based and energetically-based diseases between which they are unable to differentiate. They tend to "follow" a case, in which they are seeing where it is leading them in terms of both treatment and progress. In the case of physically-based disease, this is a prudent course to follow as it serves as a means of monitoring the healing process.

On the other hand many common health concerns are not physically-based, leaving the physician relatively clueless about the cause, so they follow along hoping their treatment measures will prove effective...which they usually do not, at least, not in effecting a complete solution to the problem.

Third, read this book and the (yet to be released at the time of this writing) Treatment Manual, and learn how to take care of yourself or find someone who has learned these methods and who will help you with your problem. The keys to a successful outcome to many difficult health problems may be found in these pages. Being a physician myself, many of my patients have found this method to be too simple and direct for them to understand how it worked.

The reason I am releasing this information in this way is that it is so simple and easy to find relief and/or gain control of many serious health problems that, once their nature is understood, the healing is the easy part. In my opinion, it is against the Laws of Nature to place this knowledge in the hands of a restrictive few while the sick and ailing continue on with their diseases. The concepts can be difficult to grasp simply because it is foreign to the mind trained in physical sciences, but the healing protocols are simple to apply.

It's time to hopefully broaden your perspective and incorporate some philosophies you may find foreign to your usual way of thinking. These are philosophies and techniques that are both new and thousands of years old. Mainly, the new part is how we will be using the old systems, to heal even new diseases. Some of the diseases we will address more directly later on include: Fibromyalgia, carpal tunnel syndrome, diabetes, menstrual cramps, PMS, Crohn's disease, migraine headaches, scoliosis, irritable bowel syndrome, anorexia nervosa, asthma, and others.

The reasons these diseases are so readily managed by the Easley Energy Therapy system (EET) is due to their underlying cause. (EET is a much simpler form of electro-meridian therapy than traditional acupuncture and uses no needles.) The cause is a problem with the energies that are being supplied to the tissues and organs, not a problem with the misbehaving tissue or organ itself. These are what I call "energy-based diseases". A physically-based health problem is typically an infection or injury. In this culture, we classify most diseases by their effect, not their cause. With this reversal of logic we tend to approach healing in a manner opposite to natural order.

What this means is that with physically-based disease, the cause and effect are both direct and proximate on a physical and historical basis; i.e. "I fell down and broke my leg yesterday." With the energetically-based disease, this physical and historical relationship is not evident, and therefore, the cause appears remote from the effect if comprehended at all, and the results is that the practitioner, out of necessity (ignorance) treats the symptoms, not the cause. There are two 'causative factors' in disease, physical and energetic, but the energetic is a mystery to conventional practitioners and these energetically-based type of diseases are very, very common.

Generally, these two different types of disease are not combined except sometimes in cases of trauma. Trauma involved kinetic energy which affects other energies. These two very different types of health problem actually reside on two different dimensions, one physical, one non-physical but having a profound influence on the physical.

As you progress through this book, keep an open mind. Much of the underlying mechanism in both the cause of the disease and the method of management are so simple that the human consciousness, which has been trained since childhood to think in complexity, skips right over these crucial bits of knowledge and concepts without notice. Often, the most profound meaning can be gleaned from the simplest of concepts.

Since Ancient Eastern philosophy is, in part, the source for some of the ideology contained within these pages, the question may arise as to whether one should memorize and thoroughly understand the intricacies of Chinese Traditional Medicine and acupuncture. To properly address that consideration, there are several answers.

First, it depends upon your goal. If one is going into Traditional Chinese Medicine as a serious study, the answer is yes – pursue your goal into that complex and wonderful world. If that is not your goal, then no, a thorough understanding of Traditional Chinese Medicine is not required.

The best answer could well be "maybe", and its corollary, "that depends." The reason for these unusual answers in that in this instance requirements to become a professional vary from one practitioner and discipline to another and one geographic region to another to such an extent that the answer must be open to those individual requirements posed by each practitioner. The basic reason for this book is to enable the interested reader to understand how the entire human being works on a practical basis without going into such detail that a whole new doctorate level of study is required, hence the "middle of the road" level of intensity of this book.

In the companion to this volume, the Easley Energy Therapy Treatment Manual (still to be released at the time of this writing), the treatments are set out in such a way that anyone with an 8th grade education can use the treatments for their own health and for their family. However, if you wish to use these treatments with the public in a clinical manner, additional education is essential. It is to the health care professional who would like to incorporate these techniques that the majority of this volume is written.

FOOD FOR THOUGHT....ACTUAL THOUGHT, NOT 'COMMON' THOUGHT

PERSPECTIVE CREATES PERCEPTION

Perspective creates perception,

Perception creates belief,

Belief creates behavior,

Behavior creates experience,

Experience creates reality...

And, our Reality creates our perspective.

It is a Circle – the Circle of Life –and the Circle of creating our own understanding of the world. It is also the means by which we create God...or at least what we think God is or does. It is also learning by trial and error, where experience is the teacher. Experience can be a hard and cruel teacher, but a teacher nonetheless. In short, by participating in this type of "logic", we are chasing our tail. When we allow others to do our thinking for us, then, figuratively, we are chasing someone else's tail, which can create an unhealthy dependence. Take the time and do the work to develop your own perspective.

With a little thought it is not difficult to understand that nothing physical can exist without a basis for that existence. Since everything physical is made up of molecules, which are made up of atoms, which functionally consist of positive, negative, and neutral electrical charges, the understanding that even physical matter is actually energy becomes evident. What is left to understand is the organization of the energy into physical objects and how they affect each other, which creates behavior of physical matter.

PART ONE

WHAT ARE HEALTH AND DISEASE?

To begin with, it would be helpful to provide the classic definitions of health and disease. It is important to keep in mind that there is a lot of undefined middle ground and much that has not been included, which include the energetic and spiritual aspects of both health and disease as they are covered elsewhere in this text.

Dorland's Medical Dictionary defines health as: "A state of optimal physical, mental and social well-being," and not merely the absence of disease and infirmity. Holistic Health is therein defined as: A system of preventive medicine that takes into account the whole individual, his own responsibility for his well-being, and the total influences - social, psychological, environmental - that affect health, including nutrition, exercise, and mental relaxation.

Dorland's defines disease as: "Any deviation from or interruption of the normal structure or function of any part, organ, or system (or combination thereof) of the body that is manifested by a characteristic set of symptoms and signs and whose etiology (history/cause), pathology, and prognosis may be known or unknown."

To clarify what health is, you must feel great on all levels. Not only must you feel great, but you must be functioning in a balanced and efficient manner even on mental and emotional levels. While the disease definition does not appear to include the entire being, it should. The health definition is more complete and accurate. Anything contrary to it in any way can be considered as a disease state. Disease usually starts in the energetic level of our being.

Upon further development, the imbalance progresses to the mental and emotional part of us; and others may start to complain about our behavior. We usually become fatigued or depressed or both, along with a long list of less common problems. By this time, the physical symptoms may begin to appear. Interestingly, it is these subtle warnings that usually go unheeded by our insensitive culture. It's not that we aren't tough enough.

It's that we are not heeding the warning signs because of other people's opinions. Sure, it is by the feedback that we get from those around us that gives us a sense of how we are doing and where we stand in the world. In the usually unquestioning acceptance of the opinions of others, often those closest to us, we forget that we are not others, but ourselves. By doing this, we just turned off our first and second levels of disease sensitivity and recognition. We are taught to ignore these alerts because of the influence of others.

In terms of the creation/development of the true physical disease state, we have just propelled ourselves to the brink of long term problems. If these beginning levels are not properly addressed, even the many physical remedies when properly applied, may not be adequate. Don't worry about being a sissy. Remember, it is your problem; and you are the one who has to manage the consequences. Those consequences are real, and they are yours.

If this sounds like mind over matter, that's right, it is. If you use your mind properly, the influences that result in disease are neutralized before they can develop into a manifest problem. In addition to that, when the mind is in proper balance, the emotions, the real movers of this universe, also behave in a healthy manner.

Both disease and health, like anything else that has been created, begin in the mind. Just as an engineer conceives an idea for something, then he designs it and draws up the plans, these are then sent to the workers who finally make a physical object out of it. If there are changes to be made, it goes through the same process for the alterations. The engineer (the mind) makes the changes, and it again goes from a concept, to a drawing, and then to the workers (the emotions) who produce or reshape the object according to the new design (the physical object). I know that many of us get the cart before the horse by letting our emotions lead our mind in the decision-making process, but look around and see how many of us are really as healthy as defined above.

HOW DISEASE PROGRESSES INTO PHYSICAL BEING

Since most of us are insensitive to the process, we develop a problem and then say "Where did this come from?" "How did I get this?" Once the energetic mold is set, the disease exists.

After all of this happens and we realize that we are in trouble, a doctor is consulted. We are informed that we have such and such disease and that we are to undergo whatever treatment is prescribed. Now the disease has become a definable reality. So, what is a disease now? Reality says you already have it; and medical science says that you must have objective findings, which means that it must be both physical and/or identifiable by another person utilizing prescribed physical or chemical criteria.

Now we are at the stage where the physical body is altered in appearance or function. This produces what is called objective findings. Now it's a REAL disease easily observed by others. Of course, it is no more real than before, only that it is now more developed.

To help in our understanding of the process of manifestation, let us consider how all of this, both health and disease, can become what they are at this point. At first this may sound radical, but we are using very simple terms and a particular point of view. Everything is created...health, disease, changes, healing - all of it is a result of creation. You don't create health by eliminating disease. If this sounds confusing, refer back to the definition of health.

Part of the key is that any change constitutes a creative process. Even a cell's dividing is a creative act. The rest of the key is that balance is the goal. At the balance point between health and disease, if you understand the mechanisms of the process, you have the choice to create either health or disease. This choice controls mechanisms of the health/disease process which may be either conscious or unconscious in its effect.

Allow me to paraphrase an old saying: Ignorance of Natural Law is no excuse. This is because it is always in effect anyway. This must be considered from a certain perspective, a very simplistic one; as almost everything is a combination of very simple steps. In this step, we consider any change a creation of another state of the condition. Creation can work both ways, positive and negative. The reason for this is that when there is no judgment, no good or bad, it just is, when it comes to the levels of functionality upon which creation is founded.

Creation is far too simple a process for opinion or judgment. Therefore, the function of creation is occurring when there is any change at all. Since everything is energy, there is no health or disease basis to work from. Energy isn't good or bad, healthy or diseased; it's just energy. When it is compared to something else, then it can have either beneficial or detrimental effects in relation to, or upon, that with which it is being compared. It is something like cooking. The ingredients are not bad or good; they are just ingredients. The meal is considered good or bad according to the combinations or methods used in the cooking process.

The same goes for health and disease. You can increase, decrease, or change either by adding or subtracting the various energies that compose the condition. It is the process of creation, that alchemical blending that is so simple and primordial that it is beyond human understanding. We do have quite a bit of control over this whole process, as we have an immense amount of control over the various components of the energy soup that we are preparing.

Every thought, emotion, action, choice of food, choice of herb, choice of treatment, choice of avoidance, etc. are within our control; therefore, there is control over the continuum of health and disease. If we don't have the knowledge to manage the recipe, it can be obtained through consultations, books, and other sources.

WHAT ARE THERAPEUTICS

The world of therapeutics is a broad one. The definition of therapeutics is simply: the science and art of healing. This brings us back to healing, what it is and how it is done. In short, healing is the moving of one's condition along the continuum between health and disease farther toward the health end of that spectrum. What healing is, in general, is Creation's influence on that which is being healed; but how people believe it is done has filled many volumes.

Therapeutics are how healing is facilitated. There are many, many types of therapies. They range from hypnotism to electro-therapy to physical therapy to X-ray therapy to massage therapy to surgery...which should be the last resort.

There is waving a burning herb over specific body parts to dipping flowers in water and ingesting that water. There are herbal preparations that are used in a wide variety of ways, and there are medical/chemical therapies. The latter is what our modern society has become most accustomed to. In fact, we have come to expect so much from medicine, usually made in laboratories from petroleum, that we and our medical professionals have lost almost all sense of the vast array of natural modalities that are available to us for many health concerns.

More than that, our scientific institutions have narrowed their scope of thought to considering that if a disease does indeed exist, it must have its origin in the realm of chemistry. Genetics has recently crept into the equation, but that too has been reduced to a combination of chemical components. As long as we stay stuck in this limited view of the way in which disease is managed, we will remain ignorant of the ways in which to apply therapeutics effectively for the areas of health concern for which we currently have ineffective solutions.

In this book, we will introduce in a practical fashion a new energetic therapy called Easley Energy Therapy (EET Therapy). The philosophical basis will be discussed; and a practical section is included. A complete with a "how to" segment to treat various conditions commonly found in our society can be found in the companion volume, Easley Energy Therapy Treatment Manual (yet to be released at the time of this writing). Most of these conditions have the distinction of being treatable (this means you can go to your doctor, and he/she will prescribe a medication or exercise that may make the condition more tolerable) but not really curable.

For clarification, to cure something means that the therapy utilized worked; and now the condition is gone. I don't mean simply suppressed or lessened, but gone. This means no further treatment is necessary, because there is no disease to treat. The term "treatment" implies no cure.

I know that this is becoming a foreign way of thinking in our society due to the vast array of health conditions that we see all around us that require long term or lifetime care (an industry goal). What this means is that, by using the conventional means of treatment, the disease is incurable. When one broadens their view of what therapeutic modalities are actually available to them, they often find that the condition in question rapidly responds to the appropriate treatment.

What is required for this proper choice to be made? First, an understanding of the basis of the disease is necessary. Next is an understanding of how the intended therapy actually works. The third factor is having the knowledge of how to apply or use the therapy, once the basis of the disease and how the therapy works is arrived at.

Often this requires quite a lot of sorting through the vast number of choices of treatment available. When we ask the average practitioner of alternative therapies, we usually get an opinion that is not only limited by their knowledge, but we are informed that this will work for that particular condition. Sometimes we encounter a little over-confidence in what little knowledge we actually do possess. This makes finding the appropriate therapy a gamble, and one can spend a very long time and a great deal of money searching for the key to their illness.

All of this usually transpires after the conventional, chemical route has been exhausted, along with one's insurance coverage, money, hope, and possibly many years of their life. Furthermore, the condition is most likely progressed to a more serious level and become more complicated by the time the appropriate therapy is discovered. Often it is that difficult to find what one really needs when one does not have a purely physically-based disease. By the way, these purely physically-based diseases are usually infections or injuries. Many of the others have an energy basis as their origin and thus require an energy-related therapy to be truly effective.

EASLEY ENERGY THERAPY

(EET THERAPY)

After a long period of being unable to come up with a name for it, I decided to name it after myself. EET is a simplified system of the art of acupuncture, without the use of needles, along with a touch of applied kinesiology philosophy that utilizes the acupuncture meridian system in both a diagnostic and therapeutic way. It is the art of determining whether the problem is entirely energetic, entirely physical, or partially one or the other, what is the dysfunctional energetic component of the recipient's system, and then discovering how to correct it.

The area of pain is palpated, that means physically touched to assess the pain; and the practitioner then determines from the location of the pain and his/her knowledge of the acupuncture meridian system which meridian is closest to the painful area. The practitioner then touches, with intent of stimulating energetically, key acupuncture points along that meridian. When the appropriate points are activated, the pain will become less or disappear entirely. This is the case of when the meridian is too empty or underactive, which is usually the case. In the case of an overactive or too full meridian, the pain will not lessen and may in fact become worse.

In this instance, the practitioner should activate an acupuncture point on the overflow meridian which will sedate that meridian, typically the sedation point. Another method is to activate a tonifying point on a meridian which is, according to the ko cycle or the destructive cycle, intended to reduce the energy in the affected meridian. Tonification is the adding of energy to a meridian. Sedation is the reduction of the energy in a meridian.

Further support can be supplied to the original meridian, if it is found to require tonification, but does not hold its status after treatment. In this case, one would provide tonification to the meridian preceding it according to the sheng cycle, the building cycle of the Chinese Element system. The sheng ko cycles are a set of energetic principles that create a dynamic balance between the yin, yang, and the five elements of fire, earth, metal, water, and wood. The sheng cycle functions to add energy to the next element, and the ko cycle subtracts energy from the next element. This forms a dynamic balance of the energies of the body, which when out of balance result in disease.

Two examples would be, in this instance, menstrual cramps and migraine headaches. With the menstrual cramp condition, one would palpate the lower abdomen, about two inches from the midline on the area of the stomach meridian. While applying a gentle pressure, just enough for the recipient to discern the discomfort but not enough to cause pain, the practitioner would gently touch/activate the appropriate points on the stomach meridian. When the proper points are activated, the discomfort will subside if the meridian is too empty, which it usually is. Of course if it is too full, the discomfort will not lessen.

Only treat the points that cause a change in the status of the problem. Every acupuncture point has an energetic character corresponding to one of the five Chinese elements of Fire, Earth, Metal, Water, and Wood. Because the various points individually each contain the characteristics of all of the other meridians, it makes sense that you cannot stimulate them randomly. The points on a specific meridian, as you progress along the meridian, cycle through the various elements in the same sequence found in the sheng cycle.

In other words, some will sedate, some will tonify, and others may have no discernible effect. This is done by touching the point while also testing the alarm point of that meridian. That is why this system is so useful to the practitioner who has not had many years of education, experience, and is not highly skilled in pulse diagnosis. Anyway, this is often faster; and as they say, the proof is in the pudding. This means that if your trial point is helpful, there is more than a passing chance that it will be of significant benefit to the recipient. Simply put, this means that you can develop your own protocol for any problem, on anyone, and at any time without having to look beyond the meridian chart on the wall or the acupuncture doll on the desk.

The times that this does not apply is when you are working on an individual that has had problems so severe and for so long that it has become so entrenched and entangled in their system that their system is too confused to manage such a simple remedy. Another is in the case of fibromyalgia. It is the equivalent of asking a simple question of someone, and they complicate it with so many qualifications and conditions of terms that you wish that you had never asked the question in the first place, because it just doesn't matter anymore. The other person's complications were so great that the question was simply lost in the shuffle.

The same happens to the being's energy system. There are other times that this basic system does not apply, but usually those are cases for an experienced professional highly skilled in this type of healing art.

In the companion to this volume, the Easley Energy Therapy Treatment Manual (still to be released at the time of this writing), the treatments are set out in such a way that anyone with an 8th grade education can use the treatments for their own health and for their family. Although the language of this volume can be complicated, and the concepts difficult to grasp, in actual application it is a simple treatment. Please do not allow the clinical language of this book to deter you from taking care of your own health using these treatments.

However, if you wish to use these treatments with the public in a clinical manner, additional education is essential, and it is to the health care professional who would like to incorporate these techniques that the majority of this volume is written.

CLASSIFICATIONS OF DISEASE, THE TWO MOST BASIC TYPES OF DISEASE

There basically are only two major classifications of disease: Physically-based disease and energetically-based disease.

We'll start with the physically-based diseases specifically for the purpose of demonstrating how limited they are in the population when compared to the energy-based diseases.

Physically-based diseases include injuries, such as cuts, broken bones, sprains, and the like; also physically-based are infections and contagious diseases. Of course, we can't forget the degenerative diseases, many of which have both physical and energetic origins in combination, like arthritis. Then there are the poison/toxic diseases that result from getting too much of a bad thing, like alcohol, drugs, etc. along with their chemical and energetic addictions.

Less common, but profound in their manifestation, are the genetic diseases. There are problems that require a cast, an antibiotic, physical therapy, pain medication, or tolerance. Usually, when they are healed, they are healed. If you get a kidney infection, you take antibiotics for a time; and when the infection is gone, you stop taking the drug. Bones heal, etc., and the cast is taken off and not replaced.

Now, let's name some common diseases; and we'll see if they are physically-based or not. Examples include asthma, fibromyalgia, diabetes, scoliosis, anorexia nervosa, irritable bowel syndrome, Crohn's disease, menstrual cramps, hot flashes, premenstrual syndrome, seizures and epilepsy, breast pain and tenderness, migraine headaches, and a large number beyond these. I'm sure you would agree that these are common problems. They are, in fact, energetically-based diseases.

Where is the infection, the injury, the genetic mistake? Are they curable? Certainly they are curable but not by conventional physical or chemical means. Are they treatable? They are to some degree depending on the condition and treatment rendered.

Energetically-based diseases have a different origin. They begin in the non-physical levels of our being. They have mental, emotional, and other energetic components. The closest to the physical level is found in the acupuncture meridian system. You basically have to go into the spiritual philosophies of the Far East to obtain a detailed description of these more subtle levels of our being.

For our purposes here, we will limit ourselves, for the most part, to the meridian system which is more or less electrical in nature. It acts much like a computer control system of the body; but it relays its information, especially in the case of pain sensations, directly to the mind.

This is what I call non-physical pain. It is not mediated by the nerves, as it does not course along the same pathways as the nerves themselves do. The pain we feel physically is transmitted by the nerves to the spinal cord and brain. The interesting thing about the brain is that it simply processes information.

Most people, including our finest scientific minds, believe that the brain senses pain and thinks. Basically it is a computer and presents information to the mind for interpretation and decision-making. Another path to the mind is via the acupuncture meridian system. This energetic network can carry information much the same as the nervous system, but the difficult part is being able to tell the difference between the two.

Since it is the mind that interprets the information from both, it doesn't differentiate between them. A pain is a pain -- period. The pain experienced in diseases that are entirely comprised of symptoms of pain, such as fibromyalgia, present an insurmountable challenge to the doctor of the physical diseases. The reason it is insurmountable is because the cause is not within the conceptual range of the physician. He/she keeps thinking nerve, muscle, bone, viscera, infection, physical damage, insanity, etc.; and so the prescriptions keep on coming, and no real cure is realized.

This is a good example of why it is important to be able to not only tell the difference between energetic and physically-based diseases but know that the energy-based diseases even exist at all. Not only is that of value, but many of our common diseases are energy-based; or at least, the key is within the energy realm. Any disease that has no known cure, is mysterious in origin, and is not the obvious result of an accident or infection may very well be energy-based. Examples include fibromyalgia, diabetes, irritable bowel syndrome, Crohn's disease, scoliosis, menstrual pain, flooding, and irregularities, anorexia nervosa, asthma, and many more.

The physical body creates the disease state in accordance with the energetic blueprint that has been created, either consciously or unconsciously; in any event, these changes can be extremely painful and destructive on the physical level. This causes quite a bit of confusion, and treatment measures are instituted that do not address the cause; and the disease, therefore, becomes incurable.

If the first two phases of the disease were properly addressed, the physical symptoms of disease would never be able to manifest. Therefore, it is paramount that the appropriate energetic, diagnostic, and curative measures be employed; as this changes the prognosis of the disease from incurable to curable.

DIFFERENTIATING BETWEEN THE TWO BASIC TYPES OF DISEASE, PHYSICAL AND ENERGETIC

Differentiating between these two is the very first part of an evaluation and the most important. Mistaking either a physically-based condition for an energetically-based one or vice versa, leads to predictable failure, hence the sorry state of health care as it now stands. This is simply due to the absence of the incorporation of energetically-based disease and treatment philosophy in the health care community at large.

A multiple approach to addressing a condition seems to be the best. This approach includes: patient history, the practitioner's training and education, conventional diagnostic techniques and testing, treatment history and effectiveness or ineffectiveness, logic, electrical evaluation of meridians, and intuition.

To put this more clearly in perspective, the following lists may be helpful. For a more complete list, please see the Appendix.

Physically-based disease:

The onset is usually known in both how it took place and when, and there is little or no vagueness to the history of the problem; upon diagnosis by several practitioners, all are in agreement; the treatments recommended are nearly identical; the time estimate for recovery is consistent; purely physically-based (example: a cast is applied to a broken bone, an antibiotic is used for infection). Energetically-based methods are not very effective, with the exception of a proficient Pranic Healer, physically-based methods are effective; the emotional status of the sufferer makes little change in the intensity of the problem; and changes in body position often result in changes in the intensity of the problem.

Energetically-based disease:

The onset is usually unknown, and how and when it began is a mystery, and there is a great deal of vagueness to the history of the problem; upon diagnosis by several (conventional) practitioners, they are not in agreement; the treatments vary due to their variance of opinion; recovery is not rapid or predictable; physically-based treatment is ineffective and, at best, provides only temporary relief; and energetically-based treatments have a nearly immediate effect; the emotional status of the sufferer results in noticeable change in the intensity of the problem; and changes in body position have little or no effect.

In the balanced patient history, the first thing normally done, unless the problem is a direct result of a physical accident, is to determine the physical or energetic-basis of the case in the beginning stages of care. When taking the history, the aware practitioner will be quickly alerted to the nature of the problem by the character of how it all began. In the physically-based case, the problem is usually well understood by the patient. They will know nearly exactly when and how it happened.

Usually, it will be the onset of some infection, an accident, or some physically-oriented occurrence that was both conscious and memorable. If the person has been treated by other practitioners, both the diagnosis and treatment patterns will be both similar and the outcome predictable.

The character of the energy-based problems is vague, the origin is usually unknown, and the problem most often manifested gradually; and the previous attempts at treatment were probably met with ineffective treatments and differing diagnoses from one practitioner to another. The exceptions to this are those problems that have been with us for a long time for which "treatments" have been developed but not cures.

Practitioners of the chemical and surgically-oriented treatment arts, while very intelligent and highly skilled, are often unaware that energy-based disease even exists. On the other hand, practitioners of the more subtle-healing arts, who primarily are involved in meridians, run the risk of mistaking a physically-based disease for one of an energetic nature. Having both the former and latter types of education and training are essential to gaining a firm grip on the greater spectrum of maladies suffered by our population and rendering appropriate care.

The previous paragraph brings to mind an example that would be well to take note of. A woman came in for treatment with exquisitely severe pain on both sides of her spine that radiated from her buttocks to the back of her head. Her family physician, not being a spinal expert, had sent her to the hospital where she received drugs – pain medications – which were ineffective. Out of desperation, she sought further help with a non-traditional practitioner, a chiropractor.

Chiropractors are spinal and nervous system specialists but not normally trained in energy-based philosophy. Had this particular doctor of chiropractic not been educated in the energy-based philosophy of healing, treatment would not have been successful due to the physically-based nature of their training and education.

The key to this case is there are no nerves, muscles, or bones that could account for the large areas of her neck, back, and pelvis that were affected; but there was an energy channel that did traverse all these areas of pain, which illustrates the importance of a more complete education, training, and philosophy. The character of the pain was also inconsistent with physically-based conditions, as it was so very painful that the slightest touch would elicit terrible pain. She did not know how she acquired this pain but had it nonetheless...a mystery so to speak.

The doctor energized the sedation points for the meridian in question, and the pain was reduced almost immediately. After sedation treatment of these meridians, she was much better – bewildered, but better. The reason for this explanation is that simply being a practitioner of one philosophy or the other is often insufficient, but being proficient in both is ideal. This is where the training, education, history taking, effectiveness of past treatment (part of the history), and intuition of the practitioner coalesce to form a useful tool to be carefully applied. In her case, physical problems were not the issue, but the problem was purely energetic in nature.

Physical tests, chemical lab work, X-rays, biopsies, etc. do not reveal pathologic results in most energetically-based diseases. The only exceptions to this are long-standing problems such as old cases of Crohn's disease and diabetes. The mechanism responsible for this is that the physical tissues receive their life-giving energies from the energy system – the energy body. This constitutes a "downward flow" from Creation to the created; therefore, without the life-sustaining flow being in proper order and character, but corrupted, the tissues degrade by the simple but profound laws of nature. These energies affect the behavior of the tissues, not their function, hence the appearance of disease, not the physical manifestation of disease.

Physical diagnostic techniques include, but are not limited to, physical exam, blood pressure, weight, X-ray, MRI, blood tests, urine tests, and other such testing one might currently find in a clinical or hospital setting.

Energetic diagnostic techniques include, but are not limited to, electrical evaluation of the acupuncture meridians, pranic healing scanning, intuition, applied kinesiology-type muscle testing, dowsing of various sorts, Chinese-style reading various body parts, micro-current readings from the auricle (the outer ear one can grasp with their fingers) of the ear, physical examination of the ear, pulse diagnosis, computerized micro-current comparative analysis, and others.

The key idea in this is that a disease must be both diagnosed and addressed on its own dimension. The physical must be diagnosed via physically-oriented tests and evaluations and then treated by physical means. The energetic must be diagnosed via energy-oriented tests and evaluations and then treated by energetic means. Failure to adhere to these basic tenets often results in attempting to diagnose and treat a problem on the wrong dimension. It could be said that such evaluations and treatment are "out of the world in which the problem actually has its existence."

TREATMENT PHILOSOPHY OF
PHYSICALLY-BASED DISEASE

The conventional means of treating disease is what most of us are quite familiar with - doing battle with the symptoms. If there is a fever, find an antipyretic such as aspirin; if there is an infection, use an antibiotic. This is called allopathic medicine. Allopathy is a Greek term that, according to Dorland's Medical Dictionary, is applied to that system of therapeutics in which diseases are treated by producing a condition incompatible with or antagonistic to the condition to be cured or alleviated.

In this system, the common approach is to provide the patient with treatment that does the opposite of the presenting symptoms as mentioned above. A possible over-simplification of this would be a fracture of a bone. In applying a cast to a broken bone the opposite/allopathic treatment is applied. This means that where the bone should not move, it does; and the cast is opposite to that, as it holds it still. Also, if there is an acute infection, treat it with an antibiotic; if there is acute appendicitis, cut it out, the opposite of keeping it; if there is inflammation, apply cold to it. Although simplistic examples, these are very good applications of proper and appropriate allopathic treatment for physical conditions.

Now you may notice that this section is very short. Of course, there are many conditions and treatments that are purely physical for which allopathic treatment is very effective. I am by no means trying to belittle this area of healing. It is very necessary and vital and should be considered in the very beginning of any health care decision. This is the area of healing that is at the very core of acute and trauma care and rightfully holds that position.

The concern is that when the nature of the disease is not well understood, often the same physically-based philosophies and treatments are applied to conditions whose origin and nature are not well understood. The result is that ineffective treatment is rendered for a length of time, often at great expense both physically, mentally, financially, and health-wise, for conditions that are not successfully treated in this manner. There are emotionally-based diseases (depression is a good example) that are treated with drugs, antidepressants (allopathic), often successfully. The only problem is that the side effects of the drugs are often as devastating as the disease itself.

This is not what I would call a successful treatment. Sure, it gets rid of the depression by stimulating the system to act in a different way, but it generates by way of side effects other conditions. Because of that, I do not classify this as a successful cure. If you arrange your classification of cure as simply the elimination of the symptoms that define the condition regardless of other problems generated by the treatment methods, and then call it a cure, that's a definition of cure I don't buy. I classify it simply as a treatment, not only a "treatment", but one with complications, which then becomes a problem in and of itself.

Sometimes, the allopathic method of treatment is very beneficial, even in energetically-based diseases; because in certain cases, and when carefully using the opposites to balance a condition, an equilibrium is reached which results in a neutralizing of the condition. Again, I would term this as a treatment rather than a cure. This is more common when there is an energy-based disease that has progressed to the point of manifesting physical changes in the order of function in the system which was not appropriately addressed on its own natural basis and now requires this form of treatment as acute or crisis care.

TREATMENT PHILOSOPHY OF ENERGY-BASED DISEASE

Energy-based disease is a disease that has its origin in the non-physical parts of the person. This can be organized in a dense-to-subtle format. In common terms, this is what is sometimes called our energy body. It consists of everything about us that is not physical. Sometimes it is broken down into its constituent parts which are named differently according to the tradition in which the discussion is taking place. For simplicity, I will use three of the more popular formats. If this is new to you, or you already have a preference, feel free to choose the one that best suits you and leave the rest on the shelf.

First, the metaphysical group uses the terms, going from innermost to outward, astral or emotional body, mental body, and the spiritual body. Those more inclined towards the Hindu or yoga philosophies of the Far East use a physical, astral, and causal body system. The third, and probably most complete, is the one used in Pranic Healing, a system synthesized from traditions found in the Far East and developed and taught worldwide by Grand Master Choa Kok Sui from the Philippines. This system goes from physical to inner aura to astral/emotional to mental to causal. In addition to these are the health rays which radiate from the surface of the physical body and expel various toxins and negative energy.

In this arrangement, the innermost layer of the person is considered first. This would involve the emotional aspect, sometimes called the emotional body. This is the part of the individual that contains and is made up of the various forms and flows of organized energy found on that (the emotional) level of existence. These are our feelings. While not actually physical in the ordinary sense of the word, nevertheless, they are real; and we feel their effects almost every waking moment.

This level of existence is very dynamic. Think about that word, emotion, for a moment. When you look at it, what do you see at first glance? You see E-motion, energy in motion. Of course, it's not P-motion, which would be physical in motion. This E-motion has no physical form. On the energetic level, it has both form and function, just like the physical body does. Emotions have definition, activity, purpose, and cause results. They can be healthy and balanced or unhealthy and unbalanced, just like anything else in our awareness.

Just like everything else, emotions have that which rules them and that which they rule. Often you will see people do as they feel (feel, of course, is the emotional component), and what they do is usually physical. The physical does have an influence over the emotional but not as profound as the emotional over the physical. In the properly functional and balanced person, the emotional level has a ruling level (comprised of the individual's belief system), as that is the direction of the flow from Creation to created, from cause to effect. That brings us to the mental level.

I'm sure that you have heard the saying, thoughts are things. Well, they are. They have definition and exist on some level don't they? Since you already have them, it doesn't require much analysis to figure that out. They are just there; they have their form, function, and results due to their ability to function. One of the ways in which they function is to cause changes in their environment. In this case it is the holder of the thought.

Since the emphasis of this book is on the lesser understood parts of our being, the energetic parts, thoughts being energetic are an integral and functioning component of both our balanced and unbalanced states of being. If we harbor negative thoughts, it weakens us and makes us more susceptible to disease. If we harbor positive thoughts, it strengthens us and makes us more resistant to disease.

The mechanism of thought forms works through our aura, then our chakra system, and into our meridian system, depending on the point of entry. By the time it reaches the chakras, it becomes noticeable as an emotion or feeling consistent with the nature of the thought form. This determines how our being will be affected. At this stage of the process, it is easy to rectify.

As it goes deeper into the system, the physical body may become involved, usually through the autonomic nervous system. This part of the nervous system regulates the blood flow and many hormones throughout the entire body. After feeling bad and not knowing why, we usually try to shrug it off; but instead of feeling better, we feel worse and more noticeable physical symptoms appear. That's when we start looking for a doctor.

THE OVERLAP FACTOR

The overlap factor is simply that physically and energetically-based diseases usually do not have a clear dividing line. Since every physical thing is made up of energy at its most basic level, it is affected by energy. Energetic problems are not so easily affected by physical input, because it is working against the flow of creation. Creation always works from the subtle (energetic or spiritual) toward the gross (physical). Sometimes the process is very rapid, and at other times it is very slow. Working from the gross to the subtle moves against the flow of creation and in the process creates vortices in the flow which result in complications resulting in the disease process.

Often, especially in the case of degenerative diseases like arthritis, the energetic and physical components are so intermingled that they may be indistinguishable. There are pains that may feel like arthritis that respond rapidly to energetic input, but these usually are more unstable in their nature and are not the true degenerative type of disease. On X-ray, they do not show the same characteristics as the true degenerative type.

With enough energetic input, and in the right manner, a physically-based disease can be rapidly treated. When done properly, a fresh cut can be healed completely in about five or ten minutes with purely energetic techniques. A broken bone may take a while longer. A well-established degenerative disease is usually very resistant, although I have seen Masters from the Far East heal these types of conditions in just seconds.

For the general public, there are classes that can start you on your way to being able to perform these types of energy healings; but it takes a complete change of how one manages their lifestyle and habits to become that level of healer.

There are a few advanced types of energetic healing techniques, Pranic Healing being one, that can bridge the gap and successfully treat the injuries, infections, and other problems that I have earlier described as being truly physically-based diseases. I know of no truly physically-based treatment that will successfully treat a truly energetically-based disease. That's why we have so many sick people in our culture.

The effect of emotions cannot be overstated. Emotion is literally Energy in motion. The energy that I speak of is not physical energy like kinetic or hydraulic energy but a higher form of energy on the order of spiritual energy. In the book The Prophet by Kahlil Gibran, there is a passage where the question is put to the prophet of understanding reason and passion. I would term these as intellect and emotion. In essence they are the same. To quote: "Your reason and passion are the rudder and the sails of your seafaring soul. If either your sails or your rudder be broken, you can but toss and drift, or else be held at a standstill in midseas. For reason, ruling alone, is a force confining; and passion, unattended, is a flame that burns to its own destruction." A little further he writes that "God rests in reason," and, "God moves in passion." (Page 50 for you research-minded souls.)

What is being said here is that reason, in its pure form, does nothing without some motive force with which to move it. It has no power of its own. Passion, in its pure form, is pure power without any direction or means of control. Lightning is a good example, except lightning does have a direction and reason for that direction, however primitive. Lightening is pure energy in motion without any reason whatsoever save the disturbance which gave rise to it and the polarity which gave it direction. A rudder is quite useless without movement, and movement without guidance is aimless and therefore dangerous.

The way that this is applied in our daily lives is that not only do we need to balance our passion with reason, but we need to supply some passion to our ability to reason properly to be active and effective in the world. Now for the interesting (bad) part: As we are growing up and haven't yet adequately developed our intellectual and cognitive faculties, our passions are already powerful. During these formative years, we have a tendency to let our emotions lead the way; and we do and say things that are not in the best interests of our fellow human beings. Likewise, they do the same with us.

There is a solvent to reduce the effects of these activities which will require a bit of a departure from our logical subject matter at this point, but this won't take long. In all of the great spiritual books, including the Bible, it is said that we must forgive ourselves and others unconditionally and always. This releases and defuses the attached emotional insults and injuries from the past.

What we need to be aware of is that these attached insults and injuries are actual energetic formations that were accepted (or endured) by us and stored in parts of our being that were delivered with the directive of intellect (I don't use the word reason here because the events which we are discussing are not reasonable, but are thought-directed) and intention-powered (passion). These energetic formations cause an energetic irritation to our being/inner self, and our energy bodies endeavor to resolve the issues that these foreign energies present. Our energy bodies don't have a means to rid themselves of these problematic foreign energy additions.

Since they are both of similar energetic nature, they combine automatically but not completely. The energy body of the being that is thus infected tries to balance the situation out with the means it has on hand, mainly change. So it changes how it works, how it is shaped, or ceases to function as well, in an effort to work with its dilemma.

Through the Creative Process, which is the normal ongoing process by which all things move through life and that which is responsible for the manifestation of things into the physical world from the non-physical world, disease states become apparent. Forming thought into words is a good example of how simple the creative process is. This is very often misunderstood. The healing of a wound is another. Of course, having a baby is the really big one.

The concept that I am trying to get across is that anything that happens whatsoever is the result of the creative process. If it were not, it could not be created and would not exist. Once we understand this, we no longer are willing to insult, injure, or abuse one another. We strive to make our thoughts and feelings pure. For those of you who believe in reincarnation, these imbalances may be transmitted from one lifetime to the next. Maybe this explains birth defects.

The long term problem is that we have often forgotten what happened to us long ago, and the insults and emotional injuries that lie dormant within our being slowly result in a negative creation process that results in what we term disease.

A glaring example of this is cancer. It was discovered some time ago by a German physician named Ryke Geerd Hamer that cancer was an emotionally derived disease and the outward manifestation of the disease was in reality the body's attempt at healing (or balance). To back up his claim, he is reputed to have had a 97% success (that means cure, not "remission") rate in a population of over 30,000 patients. Of course, this did not go unnoticed by those who make a lot of money in relation to this disease, and he was heavily persecuted.

He was known to be able to discuss with a person, literally on their deathbed, what had happened in their past which was at the core of their emotional unhappiness. Once the key emotional problem was discovered (sometimes this would take a number of hours) and the cancer victim resolved that emotional issue, the cancer would recede; and they would heal completely. Such is the power of thought when combined with emotion.

I believe that this is where most of our energetically-based diseases originate. Fibromyalgia, carpal tunnel syndrome, anorexia, Crohn's disease, menstrual cramps, scoliosis, asthma, irritable bowel syndrome, depression, and many others are in this category. These respond very well to energetic treatment. So much so that with some of them, it is like literally switching an electrical switch off; and the problem is gone.

We have a single word to describe this emotional influence...STRESS. We had very little of these types of manifestations of disease until our society became more complex and therefore more stressed. As life became more complicated and stressful, the incidence of these diseases skyrocketed. They didn't even have names for some of them 40 years ago, and now they are rampant and destroying the very fabric of our quality of life. Modern society has created stresses unknown to our lifestyle before and now we have increases in some old diseases and have also created entirely new ones.

It is the rare person who carries no grudge, loves everyone unconditionally, and is generally and truly a happy person, and almost never gets sick. They don't have the problems listed above. They have, by their emotional nature, neutralized the disease-causing elements that have been flung at them throughout their lives mainly by using forgiveness and not accepting those negative influences due to a high sense of self regard. Please do not confuse the term self-esteem with self-regard. If someone insulted them, they would know that it wasn't true and ignore it instead of storing it for later use. Isn't that why we don't let go of those old insults? We store them for later retaliatory use. Don't do it; it's a killer...for you. It causes weight gain too.

Emotions are our key to both health and disease. They are the power. It is our balanced sense of reason and the self-discipline to incorporate that sense of reason that makes the difference and determines how, or if, such emotions will affect us. The choice is yours.

PART TWO

THE PERSON AS AN ORGANISM

The physical person is considered biologically as an organism. The body has all the things that science thinks it should have to be this. Of course it ought to, as that is where science got its information. Not only that, but the scientific community is adamant about evaluating and treating the person on third dimensional terms.

Crudely put, this means that if you can't see it with your eyes and smash it with a hammer and count the pieces afterward, it doesn't exist except in the mind. Of course, they have their specialty for evaluating and treating that category of situation...by use of psychiatrists who then relegate this area of study to the chemical aspects of the nervous system or simple chemical control of that which they do not understand. This too, is a chemically-based science.

As an organism, we are relegated to the role of simply being an animal. We can go through the taxonomy of the kingdom, order, family, and species if we want to get more specific; but that serves no purpose here. We must go beyond these limiting concepts if we really want to understand how we are created and function. Physically, organisms have a number of identifiable parts that are necessary to function as living beings here on earth.

We require water, must consume food, excrete waste, have some sort of respiratory function, a control system and distribution system, and a structure within which to house all of this stuff. I left out a locomotive system, because not all organisms have one. The higher you go in the development of the being, it normally follows that the systems become more complex, numerous, and more highly developed.

Our physical system is based on three embryological layers in our early development. As the embryo goes through its early stages of development, it differentiates into ectodermal, mesodermal, and endodermal layers.

From these, we develop the various tissue types of our physical body. From the ectodermal embryological layer are developed our skin, hair, sweat glands, cornea, eye lens, nose epithelium (the tissue which lines the inside of the nose), teeth, peripheral nerves (those outside the brain and spinal cord), spinal cord, subcortical brain (the inside part), cerebral cortex (the thinking surface part of the brain), pituitary gland, pineal gland, and adrenal medulla (the inside part of our adrenal glands).

From the mesoderm develops smooth muscle (the muscle of internal organs like the intestinal muscles); skeletal muscles (the ones we use consciously and sometimes show off); cardiac muscles; connective tissue; joints; bones; blood cells (from bone marrow); blood vessels; lymphatic tissue; adrenal cortex (the outer layer of the adrenal glands); and the urogenital organs which include the kidneys, ureter, gonads, and genitalia.

From the endoderm develops the gastrointestinal digestive tract; the lungs and tonsils of the respiratory system; and internal organs like the liver, pancreas, bladder, urethra, thyroid gland, parathyroid glands, and the thymus gland. It's so splendid a system; it's no wonder that we are fascinated with it and often think that this is all there is.

As these individual parts are organized into systems and finally into a whole perfectly working system, we often wonder how it knew to become so patently specific. What I mean is that every tissue is in just the right place, all of the liver cells are in the liver and none are scattered anywhere else in the body, there are layers of tissue between other tissues to provide lubrication and containment. There is an organ called a vaginal bursa (vaginal meaning tube-shaped) that actually grows around tendons where they course over bony areas that are like a tubular water balloon for the purpose of reducing friction. How does the body know how to do that? Obviously, it goes beyond the physical body's organizational means.

The nervous system is so capable that it has been postulated that it would take a computer a city block long, wide, and tall to manage the brain's functional capacity. Of course, that was in the 1990's; and now it would only take a computer that would fill a cube with all dimensions of one hundred feet each, given the advances of our computer technology. The spinal cord is about the diameter of one's little finger. The various nerve fibers that carry the information along its length are of differing diameters due to the fact that thinner fibers transmit a message slower than a thicker one.

This system is so perfectly developed and engineered that if all of the fibers were the same diameter, the spinal cord would have to be three feet in diameter to manage its functions in the same way. Imagine if that were the case, there would be a lot more people concerned about their waistline. Just the spinal cord itself would be more than twice the width of the average person.

Physically, we are amazing creatures. If all of the sacs in the lungs were spread out flat, the surface area would be greater than that of a tennis court; and if all of the genetic material inside our cells were strung out and tied end to end, there would be a thread long enough to encircle the Earth and the Moon, including the distance between them and have enough left over to tie a large bow.

As an organism, we are truly amazing. The problem is that we are so much more than an organism, and we don't realize that this is the greatest blessing we could have.

THE STRUCTURE OF THE ORGANISM

(PHYSICAL ANATOMY)

Instead of going into a lengthy anatomy lecture, we will simply acknowledge the system on a primary level. It is important to know some anatomy as that is how many diseases are described and categorized.

The skeletal system is the framework of the physical body. It is composed of a large number of bones and joints. Most of these are in the hands, feet, and skull. Bones seldom hurt unless bruised or fractured; as they have no nerves except in the periosteum and endosteum, the layer of tissue which covers the outside and inside surfaces of bone. Bones have inside them marrow which is part of the immune system and produces the blood cells, both white and red.

Bones are actually very dynamic in their inner workings, as they are constantly being dissolved and rebuilt by cells specifically designed for that purpose. These special cells are controlled by hormones from the thyroid and parathyroid glands and serve to regulate the calcium levels in the bloodstream. There are other factors that affect blood calcium, but these are an important part of that regulating system.

One of the major concerns people have about the skeletal system is a disease called osteoporosis. This is commonly described as a disease of mineral loss in bone attributed to a calcium deficiency. While this is partially true, there is much more to this disease than that. When there is a severe mineral loss in the bones of children, the disease is called rickets. In adults, it is called osteomalacia. In both cases, the bones actually bend; as they don't have the rigidity to maintain their proper shape. The reason they don't break is because there are a large number of protein fibers in the bone too. These are made of collagen, a simple protein that requires vitamin C for its production. A chronic, severe deficiency of vitamin C causes a disease called scurvy.

Getting back to osteoporosis, there is more than a calcium loss. There are also phosphorus and magnesium losses. For bone to form and function properly, these three minerals must be in proper balance. There is still a missing factor...the protein. Why don't the bones bend instead of break in osteoporosis? It is because there is also a protein deficiency. All of the minerals and protein are in short supply. This means that there is not only a mineral availability problem, but there are hormonal and nutritional problems as well.

Poor food choices and digestion are also involved. Even sunlight and exercise are involved. Bones, when properly understood, are quite interesting and have been used here to demonstrate how they can involve the rest of the body's systems and how important the health of the entire system is to even the relatively simple and lowly bone. And don't forget that this is where your blood comes from.

The muscles are also more than they appear at first glance. While they don't have such complicated and broad based-functions as bones, they have a unique need for calcium. Additionally, magnesium is in high demand, as it is an essential element for the production of ATP (adenosine triphosphate) which moves the calcium in the course of its work. They cannot relax without it. Not only do they provide us with our ability to move about, our musculature serves as a major stabilizer of our system of bones and joints.

The muscles are a major system of shock absorbers and pads protecting us from injury by physical contact. They are very vascular and are our greatest users of energy. One of the lesser known functions of muscles is that they, and their tendons, are key constituents of our reflex system which involves not only our nervous system but our other internal organs as well. They are related by various nervous connections and the acupuncture meridian and auricular (ear acupuncture) systems in such a way that they are involved in the lymphatic drainage abilities of certain internal organs.

Specific muscles are related to specific organs and will demonstrate weakness if that organ is having a problem. The clinical science that incorporates these relationships is called Applied Kinesiology. Many of the kinesiological reflex points are also acupuncture points. For example, if the kidneys are having a problem, the psoas major muscles will be weak. This can be tested manually and reveal a subclinical (this means below the level of conscious awareness and before laboratory tests are able to reveal a problem) condition of the kidneys which can then easily be treated before the condition becomes serious or dangerous.

The joints of the body not only provide the musculoskeletal system with the ability to move in a meaningful way; but also the nerve endings (classified as mechanoreceptors found in the ligamentous capsules that surround most joints) provide the nervous system with signals that tell the brain what is going on in terms of position and movement. These are termed proprioception (for position) and kinesthetic sense (for movement) – in common terms, where the body parts are positioned and where they are moving to and from in space.

Another thing that the joint capsules do is become inflamed when the digestive process is disturbed. If particles of food are absorbed through the intestinal wall that are larger than they should be, the immune system perceives this as a threat and goes into action. One of the areas that this action takes place is in the joint capsules, possibly in the form of toxic substances. That is why the condition commonly termed leaky gut syndrome causes joint pain. The tissues, comprising the outer parts of the joint complex, become inflamed; and the result is a metabolic arthritis.

The internal organs are important for their primary functions and more. The liver has so many vital functions (over 500) that it is simpler to mention that all food that is digested goes directly to the liver for processing and storage. It produces bile, which is stored in the gall bladder and is introduced into the duodenum for the emulsion of dietary fats. Bile also buffers the stomach acid so that the small intestine doesn't get digested in the process of the food being transported into it for further digestion.

The liver is involved in the immune system and purifies the blood. It is the largest internal organ of the body and also the most regenerative. Of course, for this regenerative activity to take place, the liver must be relieved of the conditions that caused its original problem in the first place. After that requirement is met, then optimum conditions for purification and regeneration should be instituted and kept in place over the long term. The muscle related to the liver is the pectoralis major.

The pancreas not only provides the hormone insulin for the uptake of glucose but produces various digestive enzymes. The muscle related to the pancreas is the latissimus dorsi. The pancreas is located in the upper abdomen in the inside curve of the stomach.

The stomach is fairly well understood by the general public. It is located under the left side of the diaphragm up under the lower rib cage. Don't look for it down around the navel or lower, because that's only the customary place for people to describe as where their stomach is. The muscles of the neck are associated with the stomach and its health.

The spleen is on the left side of the upper abdomen just under the lower rib cage. Its functions include disintegrating red blood cells and releasing their hemoglobin which the liver converts into bilirubin. It also produces lymphocytes, a type of white blood cell, and is the largest organ of the lymphatic system.

The small intestine is responsible for absorbing digested food. It has a muscular wall which provides the peristaltic activities that move the now liquefied food along its course. It is one of the most regenerative organs in the body. It replaces its inner lining every three days. It has an immense surface area which is the result of many villi, which are small folds in its inner wall, and millions of microvilli which are microscopic projections of the villi.

When fat digestion is poor, the spaces between the microvilli become congested with fatty deposits; and this reduces the surface area to a fraction of its norm. Absorption is much reduced, but fats can diffuse through without too much trouble. It is vital to have proper fat digestion which is a function of the liver and gall bladder. The abdominal muscles are associated with the small intestine. This organ fills most of the mid and lower abdomen.

The large intestine encircles the small intestine. It has the dubious job of housing the bacterial colonies that produce our vitamins K and B12. Its main function beyond that is removing the water from its contents, so we can have a manageable bowel movement. It must be properly maintained due to the fact that the materials absorbed by it are sent directly to the liver. If the large intestine is too toxic (this is a septic organ by nature), the liver will become overloaded; and the skin, which is our largest eliminative organ, begins to help out.

This is why some people who have a diet that is rich in unnatural chemistry have acne-like eruptions on their skin that do not have the typical pus center that a typical pimple has. It is the body trying to push out something that it has no other way of managing. The muscles associated with the colon are the tensor fascia lata and hamstrings.

The heart is the most wonderful pump ever created. It does just what it is designed to do and usually without complaint. Actually, it is two pumps, a right and left. The heart has a smaller, weaker part on the top consisting of two chambers called atria. The atria are the first stage of the two stages of the pumping action of the heart. They collect the blood and pump it into the larger, stronger chambers, called ventricles; so the blood can be forced through the arteries of the body.

The weaker right side pumps blood to the lungs, and the stronger left side pumps blood to the rest of the body. In the condition called atrial fibrillation, the atria contract very quickly and out of synchronization with the ventricles and the blood flow becomes very much diminished; and the person can be severely affected. In effect, the heart becomes uncoordinated. Improper diet can contribute to this condition. The right side of the heart pumps blood through the lungs and back to the left side of the heart.

The heart is served by both the sympathetic and parasympathetic sides of the autonomic nervous system but does not depend on either one simply to beat. It has its own mechanism for this activity. The heart is associated with the subscapularis muscle.

The lungs are truly a wondrous organ. They are extremely vascular, light, and pliable. I am amazed at what punishment they can take and still keep functioning. They not only exchange oxygen and carbon dioxide but produce an enzyme that activates vitamin D, so we can absorb and use the calcium that we ingest. Of course, this also requires that we have adequate stomach acid and sunlight to get the calcium that far into the system. The muscles associated with the lungs are the deltoid and coracobrachialis.

The urinary bladder is the collection place for urine. It is a relatively simple organ but is made of a type of tissue that is not found anywhere else in the body. It is composed of a tissue called transitional epithelium. The lining isn't a muscle tissue, but it does contain some muscle fibers and contracts like a muscle. The bladder is associated with the posterior tibialis muscle.

The kidneys are marvelous. About 10% of the blood pumped by the heart goes to the kidneys to be processed. The fluid the kidneys collect is called filtrate, as it is not yet in the urine state. It is condensed to the point that only about one percent of it is actually excreted as urine. Beyond that, the kidneys have microscopic glands contained in the functional units of the kidneys called the nephron. The glands regulate blood pressure, and the nephron is responsible for reabsorbing the 99% of the fluid mentioned before. Each kidney is a little smaller than your fist. They are associated with the psoas major muscle.

The sex organs are useful for much more than lovemaking and reproduction. They produce a number of hormones which not only affect how you feel and act but how your body is shaped and where hair grows and to what extent. They determine your weight too. Beyond the foregoing, they are intimately related not only to the thyroid, pituitary, and pineal glands but to neurologic centers in the brain.

Speaking of the brain, it is the most fantastic organ of them all. Surprisingly, it has no pain sensors, so it cannot feel pain directly. The reason we feel our headaches is due to other factors. Some of these include the blood vessels in the brain which can sense pain but not the brain tissue itself. Since the brain is such a wonderful computer, we ascribe to it many attributes that it rightly deserves. On the other hand, sometimes we give it more credit than is due.

While our seat of consciousness is in the location of the brain, it is not the brain or any of its direct parts or functions. There must be a distinction drawn between the brain and the mind. The consciousness is that from which other things come, like the mind and the creative urge. It is deeply and profoundly associated with Creation. It is more of a soul thing than physical. The mind is a tool of the soul, and the brain is a tool of the mind. After that, the body is a tool of the brain. This is why there can be the existence of non-physical pain.

The mind is not physical and can perceive pain directly or through its systems that exist on dimensions beyond the gross or physical dimension. The brain processes information for the purpose of regulation and maintenance of the body. It also functions to process information and present it to the mind for interpretation. The brain can be thought of as a really, really wonderful computer. The catch is it is no different than any other computer; there must be someone there looking at the monitor to make sense of the information that it processes and presents. That is the WHO that you really are.

The brain is the driver's seat of this really wonderful organic car that we drive around for 80 or so years. We are so used to it that we have forgotten that we are even in it and have come to believe that it is what we really are. Nothing could be further from the truth. We have an energetic part of us that we use constantly. It has systems that can conduct pain to the mind directly and leave the brain out of the loop completely, and it does this so well that we don't even know the difference.

We are so well engineered that even our best and brightest physicians can't tell the difference. It is not a matter of intelligence but of conceptual awareness. Once you have the concept, the whole game plan changes; and intelligence is less of an issue. Don't let this lead you into thinking any less of your wonderful brain. It is the most advanced bio computer in the world and is barely understood by our most advanced scientists. It uses a huge amount of blood to perform its functions and is the most nutritionally sensitive organ in the system. It is associated with the supraspinatus muscle.

Now, one of the things that you should ask yourself is: Why, in a group of people that have a similar lifestyle and diet, do some people contract certain diseases and not others? Why do some women get menstrual cramps and not others? Why does one person have asthma and not another....even in the same family? Why is cancer for one and not another, and why are there different types of cancer? Why is there fibromyalgia or irritable bowel syndrome for one and not another? After all, are not their living conditions similar from a physical, chemical, and dietary standpoint?

Don't they have the same organs within each of them? Did they not go through the same cellular differentiation process in gestational development that works so perfectly that every blood vessel is the right size and in the right place? This means no liver cells in the pancreas or other confusion. That physical creative process is so perfect that it leaves little to chance. Why are there all these diseases??? It must be due to non-physical influences that can and do affect our physical being.

THE IMPORTANCE OF SYMPTOMS

Symptoms are our best friend. Symptoms tell us if something is out of order. For example, if you ate something that not only did not agree with you but could harm you, you would get sick. That is your warning to stay away from that particular item. Pain is a good one. It yells at you to go to the doctor and get fixed whatever needs to be fixed. It keeps you from overworking an injured body part. If you pull a muscle, it hurts and you don't use it. As the pain slowly goes away, you use it more and more. The pain is the controlling symptom.

They say that experience is the best teacher. Well, that's exactly what symptoms do is provide us with a guide that is directly related to our experiences if we would only look at them and read them correctly. Instead, what we do is suppress them and try our best to defeat them, so we can get on with our frantic lifestyles. What that really does for us is shorten our lives and drive the condition deeper into our being. That is when things get complicated.

Symptoms are mediated by several things. Physical mediation is carried out by the nervous system among others systems such as the hormonal system. This is common in injuries like sprains and cuts. It is also mediated by the currents of life's energy that course through the system in the form of acupuncture meridians and other channels. The chakras and aura can also mediate symptoms, although they may be somewhat more vague compared to the others.

Pain and other symptoms can be purely neurologically generated signals. Inflammation is a symptom that is normally considered chemically mediated processes. Both respond well to energetic methods, but it is still basically a chemically mediated activity.

What about pain that has no associated inflammation? There is nerve pain, but that usually has an inflammatory component. What about idiopathic pain? This means that no one knows why the pain is there. While it can really be severe and disabling, it has no physically discernible origin. This is one of the conditions that make doctors wish they did something else for a living. It is still a symptom and indicates that there is a problem that should be addressed somewhere in the system. This is where knowledge of the energy system comes in. The mind is usually directly affected without the nervous system being involved at all. The means for treatment of these types of conditions are, of course, energetic.

THE TREATMENT OF SYMPTOMS

AND IT'S EFFECT

When people have a health problem, of course the first thing of which the individual is aware is symptoms. The first thing that the doctor asks about is symptoms. The first thing that comes to mind when we have a problem is getting rid of those pesky symptoms. It is no wonder that we get caught in the trap of chasing symptoms in our quest to get well.

As we continue on our quest to rid ourselves of symptoms, we get lost in a maze of ideas, techniques, remedies, surgeries, and other myriad treatments that we hope will get rid of the pain or however the symptoms manifest.

As we continue down the path of following symptoms, the way becomes entangled both philosophically and experientially. When addressing symptoms as an entity, usually the health professional's opinion regarding the particular symptom becomes the paramount issue, overruling the opinion of the patient. This is where the ideas and beliefs of the health professional come into play. We have come to believe that the doctor is correct no matter how illogical their opinion is compared to what we think is true simply because they are the doctor, and the doctor is well educated in these things.

To address the philosophical side of this, there can be several outcomes. Depending on the specialty of the professional, their professional opinion (usually this is more personal, as it is often based on personal beliefs more than on science) may vary widely from one specialist to another. This can be more clearly seen when one presents the same symptoms to either a surgeon or an internist. The signs and symptoms of light-headedness, weakness, hunger, and sweating that accompany the clinical evidence of low blood sugar may result in the internist diagnosing hypoglycemia and advising a remedial diet; while the surgeon might deny the existence of that disease altogether and tell you to see a psychiatrist.

This has been the actual experience of some people and provides a real example. If the internist has a really effective treatment plan, then the patient is in good stead. If they rely on the surgeon and follow that advice, the consequences may not be as good; and the drugs the psychiatrist prescribes may do a lot of damage, particularly since they were not necessary and the side effects can be serious.

Experientially, what occurs is that the symptom becomes the leader in the chase for health or recovery. The symptom is the effect, therefore, the "follower" in the course of events regarding disease. If you follow the follower, in effect it is like the blind leading the blind who is following the cripple. Sort of like a reaction to a reaction, not to a cause. The indirectness of the approach nearly ensures the likelihood of failure, as the goal is not in the situation to begin with.

To be more direct, one chases the symptoms until the course of the malady results in even worse or different symptoms, which are then the new target of attention. It becomes an almost endless chase with no real goal, only the supposed goal of ridding the person of the symptom. After a while the body adapts to the situation as well as it can, and life goes on but not as well as it should have.

In our society, we have a plethora of drugs, remedies, potions, and practices that are supposed to relieve us of our symptoms. This has become a great industry, much of it protected and regulated by laws and government. This is intended to be for the welfare of the people. While it does serve that purpose, at least ideologically and politically, it also serves to protect and insulate the purveyors of these substances and practices from appropriate legal action. This has resulted in the establishment of a number of industries in the medical and health care field.

The symptoms have been the centerpiece of much of the identification of what is to be evaluated and paid for. This brings up another issue - money. As the money flows in regard to the symptoms a person develops, the stakes are raised far beyond the simple doctor-patient relationship. Insurance companies do not have the same rules as the doctors, who do not have the same rules as hospitals, who do not have the same rules as the patients, and neither has the same rules as the pharmaceutical companies. The lawyers have a completely different set of parameters, and the whole scale of things goes wildly out of proportion and completely off the subject of curing the patient which was the goal in the first place...at least from the doctor's and patient's perspective – which is the one that counts.

In short, chasing symptoms can lead the sufferer down some wild and lonely paths and still not even begin to address the problem. It gets expensive, and usually curing the actual disease in question never becomes an issue beyond the wish of the sufferer and the initial intention of the doctor. The problem is that often the doctor is symptom-oriented and goes no farther. Very often the patient is also symptom-oriented and expects no more than a symptomatic relief that they then call a cure. It is no more than killing the messenger, with the symptom being the messenger and the message sender is the disease itself – the body's response to the disease.

Still there are too few physicians in our society who consciously work for a cure; there are many physicians to be found somewhere in between when it comes to these issues of symptomatic relief and actual cure. Some actually believe the symptom and disease are the same; when in actuality, one is the cause and the other is the effect. When seen in that light, how could they be the same? Symptoms are the messenger. Don't kill the messenger; listen to him.

HOW THE PHYSICALLY-BASED SYSTEM OF HEALING WORKS

The physically-based system of healing must be, of necessity, very direct. It is a system of secondary causes, or reactions, to the initial problem that are intended to end up with a positive and desired result. The reason the term secondary causes is employed is that when an activity, such as placing a cast on a fractured limb is performed, it can be considered as a causative action. Of course, it is also a reaction to the injury; but relatively speaking, it also can be considered a cause. The reason for this is that the effect of placing the cast on the injured area is to result in an intended effect – that of causing (allowing) the bone to be in an environment in which healing will take place.

What actually happens in the physically-based system of healing is that the impediments to the healing process are lessened or attenuated, by some action, appliance, or substance under the control or direction of the physician. In the case of an infection, an antibiotic is usually prescribed. The action of most antibiotics is not to actually directly destroy the bacteria that are involved in the infection process, but to cause them to cease reproduction or impair their functioning in some way so the body's immune system can do the actual elimination of these unwanted microorganisms. In essence, the physically-based system of healing is merely placing the situation in such a position that the body's own defense and repair systems can do the actual task at hand.

THE EXPECTED RESULTS OF A PHYSICALLY-BASED DISEASE WITH A PHYSICALLY-BASED TREATMENT

Actually, the results are very good. The situation is quite straightforward and effective. It does not interfere too much with the natural order of things but in fact lends aid to natural order. This is where conventional scientific medicine is most efficient.

Physically-based disorders are very often well understood, and the methods of treatment are also reasonably well-placed and utilized. The outcome is usually predictable, and the methods are usually commonly known. One of the reasons this is an orderly process with a foreseeable outcome is that the history is easily discernible, the materials tend to be readily at hand, and the doctors and the patients can usually agree on and understand the method of management.

Without getting into exotic methods, physically-based disorders are predictable, usually not too expensive, already understood by the patient, and have a time line that is commonly known.

THE EXPECTED RESULTS OF A PHYSICALLY-BASED DISEASE WITH AN ENERGY-BASED TREATMENT

The first thing to realize about this relationship is that the two halves of the problem reside on different dimensions. They are related in a disproportionate manner rather than a parallel and proportionate manner. What this means is that the physically-based disease resides on a material, physical plane of existence. While this is quite evident, it is misleading in that there is often an assumption that the treatment effectiveness will assume a ratio that will appear proportional. The balance of physical versus energetic is nearly always very lopsided.

When a practitioner chooses a system of treatment out of tradition or training, ignoring either side of the 'human' 'being' equation and assuming only a physical basis, things won't work well. Usually, a practitioner will rely on such limited knowledge with only the good intention of trying to find the easy way out of the situation with plenty of misinformation, much of it illogical, to support these misconceptions. There is a huge difference in "density" between the physical and energetic, similar to the difference between the density differences between steam and water, but the effects of the problem (symptoms) do not reflect these huge differences, as they can be quite severe with an energy-based problem.

If one were to look at the situation from a physical science point of view, they would have a better perspective of the proportions. For instance, consider water and steam. When you boil water and form steam, it is a gas; it is still the same substance, but it requires a much larger volume in which to contain it at the same pressure and is not nearly as dense. This is where reality steps in. You must input an awful lot of steam and cool it until it condenses to accumulate any reasonable amount of water. This is an example of the transition of energy to matter.

A more violent and opposite example would be a nuclear bomb. This is where matter is converted to energy, not just a vaporous state. It has unimaginable expansive capability. The reverse of this would mean gathering a huge amount of energy to compress into itself to become matter. This is analogous to what happens when you apply energetic healing to a physical condition.

The healer must input, or channel, massive amounts of energy into the area to be healed, both properly and effectively; so it will be contained and assimilated. The more skilled and powerful the healer, the faster the manifestation of the healing will be. Not only that, but the energy must be harmonious with the purpose and the recipient. This is why great Masters can perform miraculous healings on the spot, but it takes less powerful healers considerably longer to do the same job.

Even though the treatment and disease are on different dimensions, they are on adjacent and related dimensions, which helps; and when working in this direction, it follows the natural progression of the creative process and flow from energetic to physical – cause to effect. Because of this, energy healing is relatively effective for physically-based problems. The biggest problem is that we have the mistaken notion that most of our problems are physically-based, when in reality they are energetically based.

The energetically-based diseases, through the natural down-flowing creative process, cause energetic disorders to eventually manifest as physical. In our misdirected wisdom, we think that the cause is physical when it is really energetic and has had long enough to alter the physical target within the individual's body. This is why it is possible to detect disease before it becomes a physical entity; it is created in the energy dimensions before it manifests here; and if we use energetic means of diagnosis, we can detect and evaluate these problems before the physical even notices their presence.

There are a number of these techniques available such as Pranic Healing, Contact Reflex Analysis, Kirlian Photography,

Computerized Meridian Testing, Applied Kinesiology, and many more.

The main thing to remember is to not expect more than is reasonable, and it takes a LOT of energy to condense in order to become or alter physical matter. It also takes time, just the same as it takes time for something being poured into a mould, to flow in and to solidify, only that the transdimensional transition may take longer, but it's the same principle.

This can be likened to a stream filling up a lake that is being formed. First of all, the escape route for the substance flowing in must be blocked, if there is one, and often there is. If this is not done, the beneficial substance will leak right out again. This is one of the explanations for when someone receives healing treatment and it doesn't last very long. Another is that the energy is assimilated, or used up very quickly, and more is required.

THE EXPECTED RESULTS OF AN ENERGY-BASED DISEASE WITH A PHYSICALLY-BASED TREATMENT

First of all, it should be remembered that the energy-based disease is simply on another plane of existence and not physical at all, even though they both occupy the same space physically. There are relationships and influences back and forth between the two dimensions; but due to the various "steps", or "gradations" in between, the relationship is far from being logical and direct. It's sort of a "you can't get there from here" situation, necessitating having to go to some intermediate place first. Is this logical? It may not be. Is this direct? Also, it may not be, but there is definitely a way to get there. It's sort of like going from one storey of a building to the next, in that going from one to the other is too great a distance to accomplish in a single step; but when one finds the staircase, it becomes manageable and logical.

To make matters more direct, it is just easier to dispense with the physical considerations for the moment. Once the problem has been determined to be energetically-based, use the energetic means to resolve the problem.

If one were to have a mistaken concept or opinion of the actual status of the problem at hand, thereby mistaking a physically-based problem, say, a fracture of one of the small bones of the wrist, a carpal bone, for a meridian problem, possibly the pericardium meridian, and then employ an energetic remedy. Things such as applying micro-current, moxibustion, or needling an acupuncture point along a nearby meridian, the result may be minor or may have no effect whatsoever. While this scenario has many variables, generally speaking, and since the problem and treatment are on different dimensions, they would not be congruent with one another.

It is like applying water vapor to a situation that requires liquid water or even ice. Imagine attempting to extinguish a fire with steam. It just does not have the capacity to fulfill the requirements at hand. Now, if a great enough amount of water vapor were applied, condensed, and managed, it might actually be able to perform the task at hand.

This is one of the mechanisms of how so-called miracles are performed. There is a great enough volume and a high enough quality of energy to overcome the dimensional differences. Therefore, in practical levels for "normal" health/healing practitioners, it is much more effective to apply your main efforts on the dimension on which the actual, not perceived, problem exists. Proper evaluation is of critical importance.

Usually, our well-educated health care professionals (doctors, etc.) are very good at determining what an actual physically-based problem is; it is the energetically-based problem that escapes their scrutiny and leads to inaccurate diagnosis and ineffective treatment.

Strive to understand on which dimension the patient's problem lies. Even in "mixed" examples, it helps a great deal to understand that both types of malady are found to exist within the same place and time in the same patient and sometimes in the same tissue. It becomes a two-pronged approach when this is the case.

TYPICAL ENERGY-BASED AND PHYSICALLY-BASED DISEASES, PURE AND MIXED EXAMPLES

Admittedly, this is a sticky subject. The reason for this "stickiness" is that there are so many belief systems "out there". There are so many preconceptions regarding what causes results in what diseases and the vast number of "professional" and "scientific" opinions that are so readily available through one's group of friends, doctors, almost any magazine, radio, TV, the internet, and last but not least, our educational system.

For the physical component, one should rely on their doctor, as this is the person who is highly educated in this area of concern - even though they may only know part of the story regarding any given condition. They may also present the knowledge they do have as "everything" there is to know on the subject; but often, this attitude is simply to cover up the fact that they mostly know the symptomatic and mechanical aspects of the problem.

When pushed, they will say something along the lines of "no one knows the real cause"; but they do know how to treat it. Please note that the word "treat" is used, not cure, or resolve, or put into remission; and this treatment is usually temporary unless it's a physically-based problem. Some things they will say include "must be managed" for life, but that is another sticky subject and usually erroneous.

The above-referenced information tends to create an immense amount of confusion for the lay person and professional alike. Of course, the list is incomplete, but it is surprising how many people will spend a substantial amount of money on their doctor/specialist and then follow the advice of their hairdresser, mechanic, co-worker, or even a complete stranger on their way home from the doctor's visit; and they haven't even gotten home from the doctor yet! This should illustrate how little faith people have in their physician, or probably more accurately, how confused they are in terms of what is or is not true regarding any given matter.

Generally speaking, the professional community is much more hard-line about it due to the fact that they do have at least partial knowledge about the condition. The reason for their limited knowledge is not their fault in energetic disease. Doctors are pushed unbelievably hard to get through school successfully. The reason for this is that if they weren't, they would have to go to school for a much longer period of time, so much so that it would be impractical. Anyway, it is also a conditioning process to toughen up the doctors and force them to be clear and decisive. Average people don't make it.

The same goes for nursing. The point is to illustrate the attitude of the professional, why they are the way they are, how to understand them, and what to do about the advice they give you. They are usually at least partially correct. Remember to be respectful toward them; most people have no idea of how difficult their jobs and lives actually are and what they have sacrificed in their lives to try to help make yours better. Remember that this is a subject in which they have not been trained. There is a huge abyss between spirituality or religion and science and medicine. The professional community lives on the scientific side of it.

The reason for the foregoing is simple; what follows is quite different compared to what almost everyone on this side of Asia is aware of. This list includes:

1. The physical and emotional are two parts of the same whole that require each other for proper functioning,

2. The person is first spiritual and then physical,

3. The individual is a complex of energy currents which is larger than the body, and

4. The mind can cause the body to do things which most people believe it cannot – which includes facilitating the manifestation of physical disease (or even health, for that matter).

Partial list of energy-based diseases:

Anxiety attacks

Allergies (some types)

Irritable bowel disease

Crohn's disease

Dysmenorrhea (Menstrual cramps with all of the familiar symptoms)

Asthma

Migraine headaches, chronic

Constipation (also physically-based types, if the person drinks inadequate quantities of water)

Pain syndromes after an accident that do not follow nerve pathways

Fibromyalgia

PMS

Endometriosis

Idiopathic scoliosis

Depression

Bi-polar disorder

Night sweats

Mastodynia (breast pain)

Dry eye

Painful scars long after surgery or injury

Carpal tunnel syndrome

Shoulder pain without previous injury

Tennis elbow

Thenar pain

Nymphomania/satyriasis

Frigidity

TMJ pain

Chronic fatigue syndrome

Compulsive eating disorder

Cancer

<u>Partial list of physically-based diseases:</u> (These are categorized because of space limitations.)

Fractures

Infections

Migraine headaches, usually after injuries

Contusions

Stroke

Heart attack

Genetic disorders

Constipation in the case of nerve problems or malnutrition/lack of water

Hypertension (usually dietary and lifestyle)

Arthritis

<u>Partial list of mixed energetically-based and physically-based diseases:</u>

Diabetes

Migraine headaches, common neurologically-based versus meridian-based

Cancer

Asthma of most types

Autism is still somewhat of an unknown. At the time of this writing, the best information we have is that autism is a type of energy-based disease consisting of congested pranic energy in the vicinity of the DNA that interferes with cellular function. This interference prevents the proper production of the various cellular products by overcoming the activation energy of the biochemical processes that take place in the transcription, messenger DNA production, and translation processes necessary for proper cell physiology to take place. This could possibly be in the form of sluggish removal of the histones of the DNA which would prevent the DNA from "unraveling" properly for the transcription process.

Further evidence of this as a possibility is found in the dietary difficulties experienced in the autistic sufferer along with possible reduction of neurotransmitter production, which is also evident in their limited mental and physical capabilities. The energy/physical combination explanation for this is that the complementary systems both utilize channels of ever-decreasing size until the capillary size is reached. The energetic system also does this on its own dimension. The physical and energetic systems converge at the cellular level.

There is one major difference in their characteristics at this point though; the hydraulic energy available to the blood and its kinetic and thermal energies continue to diminish until they get to the intracellular level, where they are at their lowest point. The energetic system, on the other hand, has two levels upon which it operates: volume and depth. Volume relates to the amount of energy that flows in a given area, much like water. Depth is a term that is meant to imply the transcendence of time and space due to the energetic, or spiritual, nature of this part of the equation. In other words, the equation is different in that it was due to the differing capabilities of the components involved.

The upshot of all this is that the activation energy, biochemically speaking, and the pranic or chi energy are now on a much more equal footing; and the congested prana around the DNA is now capable of significantly altering the intracellular functions on the DNA level. One more thing to throw into the mix to make it more interesting are that the neurons and other neural tissues that are intrinsically involved have one of the highest metabolic rates in the body. This is why the head requires such a large portion of the blood supply relative to the rest of the body. This simply magnifies the problem.

Of course, autism may simply be the result of the ever-increasing number of immunizations containing toxic substances being injected into children who are unable to tolerate this process as some have been saying all along.

So, what is it that makes autism such a difficult thing to understand? One is the variety of presenting symptoms; two is that children with healthy parents who live a healthy lifestyle, have a healthy mental/emotional/spiritual outlook, eat proper foods, get adequate exercise, and raise their children this way, seldom have children who exhibit autism. Now, I mean these parents actually have excellent lifestyles and not simply the absence of disease.

On the other hand, we have children who are in families that eat over-processed and manufactured food with lots of additives, use numerous medications for every little problem, engage in less than healthy emotional/mental/spiritual practices, exercise very little, and have, in general, a very poor lifestyle in terms of being natural and holistic.

Some have noted there is a distinct lack of autism among the Amish populations. This may be attributed to the reduced amount of cell phone and other radiation to which they are exposed. It has been presented by some scientists that electromagnetic radiation causes the normally non-pathologic levels of yeast and fungal populations, found in the average person, to react aggressively to these electromagnetic influences. Microorganisms defend themselves by greatly increasing their reproductive rates and their exotoxin production when they sense a threat. This has been experimentally proven to result in a 600 fold increase in the reproduction and exotoxin rate above normal when studied in laboratory experiments.

The adult central nervous system is already established and developed and is less prone to such internal assault. The brain of a newborn is not so well defended; and when this onslaught takes place, the development of the brain is not only inhibited but actually damaged. While I have not carried out these experiments myself, when one realizes the increase in these electromagnetic frequencies and the increase of the incidence of autism are on a fairly parallel course, you are free to draw your own conclusions. Couple that with the toxic ingredients of the many immunization injections children receive, particularly in that mercury is a very potent neurotoxin, it is very reasonable to conclude that both radiation and mercury toxicity form a primary team in the production of autism.

When I began practice in the mid 1980's, autism was rare; but now, decades later, it is very common as are cell phones. I believe that genetics are involved, mainly in that some children are more or less tolerant to microorganism-generated stress than others. In this time of spiritual evolvement on a physical level, it is reasonable to consider that these sensitive children who are more likely to suffer from, and be more intensely affected by, such microorganism and chemical assault, are actually inhibiting our own evolution as a species by these insults to our biology.

The above brings into view both the physical and energetic dimensions, with the energetic having the most influence, which is natural; as it is the dimension of cause and the physical is the dimension of effect - the Creator and created, so to speak. It is a natural "down flow" of manifestation. With all this said, autism is most likely a mixed disease, energetically and physically speaking, with the energetic (electromagnetic) at the forefront and as the main cause.

It should be remembered that these are partial lists, and that generalizations have been made. Please be careful not to confuse the appearance or manifestation style of the disease with the actual cause - without which the disease could not exist in the first place. We are talking about cause, not effect. If manifestation were all we were considering, the origin of these problems may never be found; as we could never leave on the journey for the destination as we would still be searching for the starting place. If you don't know where you are, how can you determine the correct route to reach your destination?

PART THREE

THE PERSON AS A BEING

"Being", that five letter word that means so much more than one might suspect. Being is quite a malleable word in the English language. Let's look at the length and breadth of this common word before proceeding due to the importance of understanding this simple word's power.

Examples: Among the various forms of energy-based treatments employed at my clinic, all of the following were treated with micro current therapy. The system used is called Easley Energy Therapy, which is unique in its simplicity and profound effectiveness. Additional energy therapies of Auriculotherapy and Ryodoraku, both micro current therapies, were sometimes used.

Due to the confusion with which this situation is normally infused regarding physical body and spiritual being (or energy body), a few examples may be useful in understanding the scope and power of both regarding the individual as a physical body and a being. The physical body is the recipient of the maladies suffered by the energy body, so when treating the energy body using the physical body as a map, amazing things can happen. Examples include: a man with the 3rd, 4th, and 5th fingers of his left hand which had been stuck in a flexed, or curled, position came in for treatment. He was told that the only hope for restoration of normal use of these fingers was an extensive surgery to lengthen the flexor tendons of these fingers. After about five minutes of applying an energy treatment to his hand, namely the component that was causing the physical hand to misbehave like this, he was able to straighten his fingers and use his hand normally.

One of the principal concepts this book is intended to convey is that the energy body dictates the behavior of the physical body. In another example a woman came in for treatment of a long standing case of fibromyalgia. She had suffered with this condition for 23 years, being bedridden for two years. After analyzing her energy system and balancing the components that were in a pathologic state, her condition was resolved. Upon contacting her for follow-up visits several times, she explained that was not necessary, as her condition was completely resolved.

In another case, while attending a convention, a dentist friend introduced me to her friend, another dentist. The friend was very thin and reported she had anorexia nervosa, to which I replied it can be resolved in short order. She told me to treat her and upon treatment, she said that she immediately became hungry and left to get some food.

A family who was under my care brought in their teenage daughter who could not keep her food down, had diarrhea, and was missing a lot of school due to this condition. Examination and history revealed her condition was energetically based in origin. Upon treatment, she was returned to normal. Two follow-up treatments were required.

A woman came in for treatment for diabetes. Using Auriculotherapy and Easley Energy Therapy techniques, her blood sugar was lowered substantially after the first treatment. After following a remedial diet, exercising (walking), and further treatment, she lost 60 pounds and went from having a blood sugar level of 428 to normal. These changes took place gradually over an eight-month period of time. A key phase of her therapy was recognizing and altering an emotional issue that had an obsessive character to it.

A senior lady came in for treatment of asthma. She came in only when she would have an attack, so this was a very crucial event. After several visits several months apart, her asthma was resolved. The main therapy used was micro current Auriculotherapy.

A lady came in for irritable bowel syndrome. After a single treatment both her irritable bowel syndrome and her menstrual problems were resolved.

A young man came in for treatment of a shoulder injury. After an orthopedic exam of his shoulder, a single reflex point was treated with Easley Energy Therapy which resolved the energy body injury he sustained at work. A similar situation took place when another young man came in with persistent shoulder problems. He had recently received a vaccination that caused a problem with the energetic part of his shoulder. Again, a single micro current treatment resolved his issue.

A woman came in with precipitous labor. She was five months pregnant and was in fear of losing her baby. Her doctor told her she would have to stay in bed for the remainder of her pregnancy. Having other children to care for, she sought other remedy. After investigating her symptoms, she was treated using an energy-based treatment, specifically micro current. Her symptoms diminished before she left the treatment room and she reported that her problem was completely resolved when office staff called to inquire of her condition.

Hopefully, these examples will serve to illustrate the importance of health care professionals, either conventional or alternative, being trained in this form of care.

In the larger sense, "being" means anything that has existence on any level or dimension. It can be used to describe God, a galaxy, solar system, blade of grass, a thought, an emotion, a thing with no consciousness or total consciousness, a germ, or any "thing" anywhere.

Now that we have that word expanded to a reasonably adequate dimension, let's begin to qualify it. What kind of being is it? Is it a human being, a bacterium, a planet? Any of these fit the definition, but what I am trying to do is bring your attention to the limitlessness of your own being. The human being is our main concern here, but it is necessary to realize that there are beings within beings within beings. In other words, we are multilayered. That goes for both the physical and energetic/spiritual components of our "beingness".

This is important, as it is this multiplicity of our parts and our dimensions that tend to make us unwilling to investigate our entire beingness due to the daunting immensity of the task. Then again, there is that eternal, insistent compulsion and urge to learn and know more about our origins and makeup. It forces us to engage in many of "life's" activities in that eternal search for "happiness" which is only found in knowing and having access and use of our entire "selves". That is what drives us to goal after goal in our search for satisfaction, only to find out when we "succeed" that we only experience a temporary respite from that eternal compulsion to be more than we were.

This compulsion is actually our constant reminder of our true "home" in the grand scheme of things – our origin. So, to address this subject properly, it would make sense to start at the beginning of the being. First, please notice how being and beginning start with the word "be." We'll let that scratch at the door of your consciousness for a while, so we can discuss where we came from and where we are going, because it is integral to what we are when it comes to being a being.

Almost all of this is related to us down through the centuries as parable, myth, religion, religious mysteries, fairy tales and folklore, to mention just a few. In the biblical sense, we are the living children of the Living God. This simply means that we are an original piece of life of the Original Life. Again, biblically, there is a passage that says "In my father's house are many rooms" (mansions in some translations); and preparations are being made for your arrival. (John 14:2)

What is not being said is that this is not only where you are going but where you have come from. It is actually the place and substance in creation where you began, never left, and to which you will return. It is the part of you that is connected to the Source of Life and from which the life that "lives you" flows, not the life that you live, which is a misnomer.

As this flow of life descends from the part of you that resides on that first level of Creation, it flows down something that we call the "spiritual cord." This is the equivalent of an umbilical cord for a fetus in a mother's womb. Through it flow the various qualities of life energy called "prana" in India and "chi" in China. In Christianity it is called the "Holy Spirit." As the flow enters the area of the incarnation, which is the place where physical matter becomes involved, in other words the physical body, it enters the top of the head at the crown chakra. This is what one might call the "trunk" of the tree of life.

From our physically-oriented perspective the roots are upward, planted in what the Bible calls the "firmament." The flow of life goes down its "concentration gradient", which means that it flows from a greater abundance to a lesser one. After entering at the top of the head, it courses down the spine and goes to the sacrum, a large bone at the base of the spine. On the way down the spine, "branches" diverge to form the chakras, which might be likened to the "branches" of the tree of life. When the flow reaches the sacrum, it is divided into four channels, or rivers, two of which wind/spiral and two of which do not, as mentioned in some translations of the Bible (see quote below). The two that wind are also recognized as the two major nadis in Far Eastern philosophy and are also represented as the two serpents on the medical caduceus, also called the "staff of Hermes". (Hermes is the messenger of the gods in Greek mythology.) The two "rivers" that don't wind are what we know as the conception vessel and governing vessel in Chinese medicine. They manage all of the yin and yang energy, respectively.

Biblically it is found in Genesis. "But a mist went up and watered the whole face of the ground" Gen. 2:6, and "A river flowed out of Eden to water the garden, and there it divided and became four rivers." Gen. 2:10.

As these channels of energy progress, they branch, becoming smaller and smaller in size until they reach capillary size – much like the cardiovascular system. The chakras act as pumps that spin clockwise and counter-clockwise alternately. This activity functions to drive new energy in on the clockwise part of the cycle and expel used up energy on the counter-clockwise part of the cycle. This is very much like inhaling and exhaling.

As the energy courses through the system, it passes through the various chakras, which condition and alter the quality of the energy, making it suitable for the various purposes the being needs at that particular juncture. This is very similar to the manner in which physical organs function. As the energy is "pumped" by the chakras, it is forced through nadis (translated from the Sanskrit word nadi, meaning "spiritual tube" or "psychic nerve"). These nadis and the meridians continuously branch into smaller and smaller channels.

There are twelve, (yes, twelve not just seven) major chakras, some of which have been kept secret for thousands of years except for only the more advanced students of the higher, and secret, levels of spiritual practice. These can be seen as the sefirot of the Kabbalistic Tree of Life, but they are also represented in many other ways. A few of which include, on various interrelated levels: the 12 two-hour segments of the day, the 12 pairs of elders around the throne of God, the 12 signs of the zodiac, the 12 apostles, the 12 months of the year, the 12 inches in a foot, the 12 chakras, and the 12 universes of which few are even able to discuss intelligently mainly due to their mystical nature. Even a circle is made up of multiples of 12 (30 multiples of 12 degrees each).

Understood properly, the above constitute a group of aspects of the same concept and are depicted on various levels of symbolic schematics. What this means is that it isn't what it looks like; rather it looks like what it means; it's just that no one ever told you to utilize this perspective when making these considerations, also which probably never were brought to mind to begin with.

The energy body, sometimes called the soul, is much larger than the physical body which more or less occupies the center of it. Actually the "soul" is indefinable because it is part of God, but we'll simply use this term for convenience. This is why, when studying esoterics, they discuss the layers of the energy, or soul body, going from inside to out as emotional, mental, spiritual, etc. This means that the more subtle parts are the outer layers. Then, going inward, we have the physical body with its layers of skin, muscle, bone, and viscera.

When it comes to the physical, we get to the point where everything comes in matched pairs of two, usually a left and right. When it comes to the combination of the physical and energy bodies, we have the mind and brain, one energetic and the other physical. Likewise, we have the chakras and organs, the vascular system and meridians, the nadis and nerves, and so on. Even the Bible says we have two bodies, one terrestrial and one celestial. See 1 Corinthians 15:40.

What has been called the "observer" is what we commonly call the consciousness (the part of each of us that resides above all the disturbance of what we normally view as 'life'). This is the part of us that is the "person behind the scenes" as if a puppeteer is operating her/his puppets from a hiding place. The outer world, including the body, is the stage, but is also an anchor to which the more subtle is attached, which helps give it meaning and orientation. It's quite a dance.

So, we are all of these things. All put together by the Master's hand for purposes that few have discerned during the history of time. We are so much more than we could ever imagine, and it is this unconscious greatness that gets us in so much trouble at times. Therefore, I place this challenge before you: Challenge this unconscious greatness that is not only within you, but is you. Prove me right or prove me wrong; but prove something of value!

You may have heard that "heaven is within" and that the body is "a temple of the Holy Spirit" among other things. Well, if this is true, why don't we all have the power to toss mountains into the sea? Because we, as beings of free choice, being the sons and daughters of the Most High, have not only free will, but near ultimate authority due to our close relationship with Creation which has resulted in our creation of our world as we see it. That is why you may have heard that we are co-creators. Not only is this true, but you cannot avoid it - you're stuck with it, so you better get used to it. Let's return back to where did the power go?

We, through our own poor choices and other distractions and mistakes, have clogged our systems to the point where we are barely functional on these levels. This means that we are "flow challenged" beings of great potential, and flow is essential to great works. It also helps to explain why we often behave more as animals than the Children of the Divine who we actually are.

As beings of such great potential, aren't there ways to access this potential? Sure, but first of all, one must be constantly aware of the fact that this physical world in which we place so much confidence is a world of effect, or result. It's a reaction to put it in a different but useful way. We must go to, and be in concert with, the levels and influences that are on the creation side of the equation of life. This requires our acting much more like a "being" (spirit) rather than a "human" (body). It is the human side of things that causes so much of the problem, but this is due to our unconscious immense power that creates continuously whatever we think and say.

We have access to the 12 universes due to our being a microcosm, a miniature version of the macrocosm, which is where so much of our ability derives, including our common characteristics such as how we feel emotionally, thought processes, creative urges, the ability to heal, to love, to think, and so on. It is all really so simple that we have overlooked it, with science there to help distract us with its own logic. So, we beings have a great deal of potential, so now how are we going to manage all this greatness toward a positive goal? With free choice…it's up to you. Since you are reading this book, most likely you are going to use it for healing, education, and self-evolution; therefore, you have a starting place.

If it seems that the foregoing is obtuse and indirect, read it a few times to let it sink in. If it were explained directly, it wouldn't make sense. In this case, it is better to describe the parts and infer the whole, rather than just blurt out something that is not readily apparent, even to the most careful eye.

With all that said, there are some other things that should be brought into the picture, such as the physical body. Ultimately, the physical body is made up of earth. Every bit of it has come from the physical planet. You may have heard that "you are what you eat and breathe". Well, it's true. What else would you be? It is the physical counterpart (physical body) that holds us still long enough to learn about life in a meaningful way, no matter how uncomfortable it may be. It is a conditioning process in which eternal habits are formed so that the higher portions of our being can evolve. Remember that perfection may imply evolution; but it doesn't; it only implies perfection – and evolution is entirely another issue.

THE STRUCTURE OF THE PHYSICAL BEING (ANATOMY)

To go into the subject of Anatomy in a detailed fashion here would be far too cumbersome and is not necessary, nor is it my intention. A description will suffice regarding what it is, but there are some things about true anatomy many people have not considered. That said, "true" Anatomy includes the energy body, while conventional physical only Anatomy does not.

Anatomy is a vast subject that basically involves the physical structure of the human body. The body has layers, tissues, and systems that are homologous (similar) to those of the energy body. Anatomy studies in a systematic manner all of the aspects of the body, usually beginning with the organization of structures starting with atoms, and progressing through molecules, cells, tissues, organs, organ systems, and finally the complete organism. When looking at the body from a layer perspective, from outside to inside, it has the hair, skin, a layer of fat, muscle, bone, and viscera.

Beyond that are the microscopic structures which are within the blood vessels, glands, individual organs, and muscles such as cells, beneficial bacteria, and the cells' inner parts. These inner components are the building blocks of the larger structures and are the foundation of their ability to function.

Each of the different tissues has its function. The same goes for the organs, muscles, and the rest of the structures. Each organ and tissue has a means of regulation and communication with the rest of the body's community of parts.

The most fascinating part about anatomy is that which I do not believe science understands in regard to development and cell differentiation. This would seem to apply especially to Developmental Anatomy, but actually it applies to all biology. Specifically, what I am talking about is the ability of the tissues to develop so exactly where they do, how they do this, and why things don't get confused in the process.

The cell differentiation theory is one in which it is assumed that, due to cellular crowding and layering during embryonic development, the cells know what to become. A convenient term "stem cell", actually quite valuable term on its own, has come into use. It doesn't actually explain a whole lot, but it really sounds good. It is a very handy term. Certainly, that doesn't answer the question of how does this cell know what to differentiate into. Of course, there are numerous chemical and biological signals in the developed system for this process.

What about early development and the production of the same tissue, such as a blood vessel or nerve in a part of the body that has been injured, as this part must replace itself? What is it that makes a nerve or blood vessel branch exactly where it does or causes the muscles to form exactly the way that they do along with their various layers of fascia separating them? How is it that a muscle/tendon unit knows where the muscle should stop and the tendon should begin? Why are the arteries found in the inner, more protected areas of the limbs rather than simply wherever is convenient? Maybe they actually are, but I just haven't realized it yet.

Anyway, when you look at the magnificent detail and the great precision with which the physical body is constructed, it is absolutely amazing. This is even more astounding when one considers that every cell in the body has the same "brains" or DNA but selects the portion of that DNA for its specific needs and purposes.

Now that I have thrown half of science's answer to these questions out the window and probably upset some of those great minds that know a lot more about this than I do and actually have solid answers to much of this, it still remains that there is an awful lot we do not know, probably much more than that which we do know. Since this book is about how the entire system functions on all of its levels together, other factors or influences must be included for a more complete understanding.

This can be called the "mould" or "form" theory. But, as I hold it as a foundational paradigm, there are not only two sides to every story but to everything that exists physically. A biblical reference is found in 1 Corinthians 15:40 indicating the two-body structure of the person. But these two bodies, one physical and one non-physical, are anchored and rooted together into a functional whole whose parts are internally intertwined.

A gardener's example would be two seeds planted in the same small container and allowed to grow to an appreciable height. When they are to be transplanted in the garden while still being individually separate, their roots are quite intertwined and difficult to separate. Is one of a higher order than the other, or does it have precedence over the other? With the example of the plants, no; they are on equal terms. With the physical body and the energetic one, there is a difference as the energetic one has precedence due to the descending nature of the flow of Life, not to mention the immortality and mortality issues.

The physical is the created one and the energetic is the creating one. Considering this, it can be seen how the energetic portion would be the receptacle for the physical portion in terms of form, because it is the energetic that is the "mould". This includes every part, cell, blood vessel, nerve, and bone - even the convolutions of the brain.

Scientifically, this is normally seen as a "concentration gradient", meaning that there is some natural "pressure" causing things to happen. This also explains to some extent where the pattern for differentiation, and sometimes physical defects, originates. Simply stated, it explains how each blood vessel knows where to be rather than to be somewhere else. Another way to say this is that our individual systems are literally physical matter (flesh) "wrapped" around an energetic form to which the physical must conform. One is within the other...literally.

HOW THE BEING WORKS (ENERGETIC PHYSIOLOGY)

As in the above section on Anatomy, it does not appropriately serve our purposes to expound on classical Physiology. One is able to consult any quality text on that subject to gain normal "scientific" knowledge in that subject. Of course, this is quite helpful in understanding the purely physical functioning of the human organism; but we are going well beyond that here.

While Anatomy studies how the physical body is constructed and what it does, and Physiology studies how and why it functions, we are discussing the "being" here, which is much more than just a physical body.

To keep things simple, we will begin with the "functioning" or "physiological" part of the being. This begins just above the physical head. Remember that we have two bodies, one terrestrial and one celestial (physical and non-physical). For every physical part, organ, etc. there is an energetic or spiritual counterpart. In actuality, just the reverse is true which means every physical part is the counterpart of the spiritual/energetic structure. The reason for this seeming reversal is that the physical world is not the "real" world. Of course, it is real; but it is the world of effect, or result. The world of cause, or creation, is the spiritual/energetic world. Sometimes it seems we humans have always done things backwards. Maybe this explains it.

There is a connection with the higher parts of our being that resembles a river of life that delivers to us our life energy. This is commonly called the "spiritual cord" in metaphysical circles. It is through this spiritual structure that the life "force" that lives and breathes us enters into our incarnated being. Again, I will explain why this is stated as such. We may have two bodies, one terrestrial and one celestial; but we also have two souls. Actually they are two parts of the same one, but they seem so far apart so much of the time. There is the Higher Soul into which the Creator and Author of Life pours the essence of life, as a parent would feed an infant child.

The life energy is then transmitted down a three-stranded cord from the higher soul to the incarnated soul, much like a physical umbilical cord going from the placenta to the fetus. The incarnated soul has its resting place in the 12th chakra, which is just above the head. The energy then courses through the crown chakra and the sushumna nadi, which traverses the spine. As it goes down, other chakras branch off until it reaches the sacrum where it splits into four heads or channels. Two of these are the ida and pingala, which are represented as the two serpents of the medical caduceus (biblically called Pishon and Gihon), while the spine/sushumna is represented by the staff. The two remaining channels are called in modern language the governing vessel and conception vessel of acupuncture (biblically called Tigris and Euphrates).

These are the four rivers that flow out of Eden in Chapter 2 of Genesis and interestingly flow out of Eden to water the garden (of Eden). The channels then branch profusely and distribute the energy of life throughout the being. These are called "nadis" in Sanskrit, which means "psychic nerve" or "spiritual tube". These are homologous to the nervous system of the physical body.

The chakras, more or less, form the "branches" that extend from these nadis. The word "chakra" is Sanskrit for "spinning wheel"; and they are called such due to their appearance resembling a wheel that spins in one direction and then the other, alternating direction quite rapidly. These are functionally identical to the organs of the body, each being located in a different place, having its own color, function, size, and character…just like the organs. They also have a relatively direct effect on the function of the physical organs. They act somewhat like vortices that process the energy and transform it for their specific purposes.

The last of the major energetic components are the acupuncture meridians. These are homologous to the vascular system of the physical body. They serve as channels that enable different types of function in the energy body in its interfacing with the physical body. Acupuncture meridians can transmit pain or block functions similar to a nerve's ability to do so. When they are disturbed, they often can alter the functioning of actual physical organs.

All in all, the energy of life flows through these energetic structures in ever-descending branches until the channels are microscopic in very much the same manner as the nervous and vascular systems.

Prayer, thought, emotions, and intentions all have a direct and profound effect on these structures because they are all on the same general dimension - the spiritual or non-physical. This is the key to understanding how "psychosomatic disease" works.

These channels radiate their life energy into the tissues of the physical body in a similar fashion as the capillaries sending out their products from the blood into the cells. It is on this cellular and DNA level where the two, the physical and energetic systems, have their most intimate interface. Imagine if you will how little interference it takes to impede the flow of blood in capillary circulation. Then consider how it would take an equally minute thought, emotion, or intentional influence to disturb, amplify, or impede the flow of life energies in these energetic channels. When an acupuncturist talks about "stagnant chi" or some other type of chi, they are describing this process.

In short, the energetic feeds the physical in the normal flow from creation to created, cause to effect. Whenever one moves the physical body, it is the energetic body that leads every movement. This is the principle of hatha yoga when performing the postures. It re-establishes and balances the flow of the energetic into the physical and conditions the physical at the same time.

THE IMPORTANCE OF SYMPTOMS...AGAIN

Repeat the following mantra three times. Symptoms are my friend. Symptoms are my friend. Symptoms are my friend. Also, a dog is said to be man's best friend; and this is said without qualification as to whether or not the dog bites.

First consider the nearsighted approach to symptoms. Imagine having a dog that lived outside your house; and every time you fed or visited this dog, it would bark, bite you, urinate on your foot, have diarrhea, or simply scare you. Also, you never claimed to own this dog, but it simply appeared in your life and would not leave until it was good and ready. Often you would not even know it was "out there". You probably thought it belonged to someone else. When it would bite you, sometimes it would not bite too hard but on other occasions, would clamp down more firmly. Please be aware that this refers to an irritation or pain, not an actual dog.

Now consider the farsighted approach to symptoms. Contemplate the above and then also realize that you live in a house in the jungle and you are part of the food chain. When you go outside this dog manages to keep away, to a very great extent that which may pose a danger to you. This is mostly a warning sign and communicator that something is out there that will eat you. Even if you experience a bite or two and if you heed the warning, you will be relatively safe.

Symptoms act as an uncomfortable, irritating watch dog that warns you of danger and barks and bites to alert you to the fact that action is necessary. The dog of symptoms only barks/bites when there is danger beyond your normal limits...or that danger has encroached into areas of your life that you normally consider "safe and secure".

This metaphoric "dog's" function is communication and warning. I know that this is a strange name for a dog; but in this case, he is your best "unfriendly friend" and will save your life if you pay attention to his more gentle "bites" before his assigned duties require him to bite down more firmly. He is trying to save you from greater danger or even save your life.

"Modern medicine", and especially the drug industry, does its best to pull this "dog's" teeth; so hopefully you don't have to suffer in the least. After years of this kind of "healthcare" your normal limits become smaller, more contracted, and brittle. Symptoms become more aggressive and your former latitude, in terms of time and choices, shrinks more and more.

Defining symptoms is relatively simple, although many people don't have a clear idea of what symptoms are, especially when considered with "signs". Simply put, symptoms are the complaints that one presents to the doctor. They are subjective and arbitrary; they provide information but usually no direct and definitive data for the physician. They do not tell you, or the doctor, why something is the way it is only that it is present.

Usually a person is not able to tell the doctor what the signs are, unless they are well-educated in this area and can provide objective information about themselves, which is usually not the case. Even then it is only limited. Signs, on the other hand, tell the doctor a lot. These are the objective findings that are determined by the doctor utilizing diagnostic techniques, using symptoms as a guide as to which techniques to employ in his or her search for why you are having a problem and what that problem actually is.

Symptoms are usually pain, discomfort, fever, a rash, something being discharged from the body, something that has ceased to work properly, etc. These are the names we give the "dog bite" of symptoms. In short, symptoms are what the patient notices and tells the doctor about, and signs are the reactions or responses the doctor causes to take place because of some test or procedure he or she is doing for diagnostic purposes.

In recent decades, our society has become distracted and unaware in terms of what is going on within itself. People used to be able to describe to the doctor when, how, where something hurt, what made it worse, and what made it better. Now, when asked about symptoms, often the patients are so poorly described, it is impossible to obtain anything other than the most general information about what it is that may be the problem.

I remember one particularly vague patient that came in for back pain that could not tell me when asked, "What part of your back hurts, the lower back, middle back, upper back, or your neck?" He did not know! This person was so unaware of his own body that he was unable to tell me where to examine him other than the back side of his body. This is equivalent to someone smashing a finger with hammer, going to the doctor, and saying "My hand hurts!" and not knowing why it hurts or even which finger they smashed.

I know that this is an extreme case (this person was not stoned on drugs, only really, really unaware), but it's becoming more common for doctors to treat people as a veterinarian would an animal which cannot communicate verbally, so the doctor may have to perform even more tests to discover what the problem is and what to do about it.

THE TREATMENT OF SYMPTOMS AND ITS IMPORTANCE

There are a number of reasons to treat a person based mainly on symptoms. First of all, the symptoms are why they are seeking care in the first place. It hurts, itches, or whatever it's doing that it should not be doing, or not doing something that it should be doing. If a doctor doesn't fix symptoms, the patient has no way of knowing if they have been helped or not.

Symptoms are a guiding signal for the physician to follow. Ideally, they will have a logical match-up with the objective results from appropriate testing, which they are supposed to help determine.

Of course, treatment based on symptoms runs a high risk of not addressing the issue that the patient requires to be addressed. If, and hopefully this is often the case, the problem is a physically-based disease, such as an injury or infection, then this style of treatment is effective. On the other hand, if treatment is not effective, this may be an indication that the problem is not physically-based, but energetically-based instead.

When treating symptoms, rather than treatment because of symptoms, the physicians often enjoy an improved public image and usually make more money. The downside to this is that often the underlying cause is left unaddressed; and therefore, the patient is, in effect, left untreated...but they feel better for the time being and will tell their friends.

The moral to this story is the symptoms are there not only as a warning to the patient that something requires attention but a pathway for the true physician to tread in order to discover the actual cause and apply an appropriate remedy. Far too often symptoms are used simply as an advertising tool for those "snake oil" interests whose only concern is profit. Pay close attention to their ads, and you may find that the side effects are worse than the disease they are intended for.

HOW THE ENERGETIC SYSTEM OF DISEASE WORKS

There are two foundational principles involved in this area of activity: the "creation gradient" principle and the "creation interference" principle.

The "creation gradient" principle is my descriptive term for the flow of energy from the higher realms of Life into this one and through the individual. Meaning no offense to anyone's philosophy, but anyone who thinks that we function and exist solely on the basis of the food we ingest is not living in the proper dream world. The Bible says that "man does not live by bread alone". One very basic interpretation of this is that something else is coming into our bodies (and probably going out of our bodies too) that is far beyond food and the physical dimension altogether.

As was discussed before, the Life Force, Holy Spirit, Prana, Chi, or whatever you want to call it, enters into us from above, travels down the spine, diverges at the sacrum, is distributed throughout our being via the chakras, meridians, and nadis in channels of ever-descending size until they reach their smallest dimension where they radiate out of themselves that Life which we receive from Above.

The operative principle of the "Creation Interference" model of disease production is one of starvation or corruption. It is a clogging of the vital channels. This results in a reduced flow of Life into the incarnated soul structure which compares to a reduced blood flow to the physical tissues. The result of this is corruption, dysfunction, and general spiritual starvation.

This affects different people in different ways. For instance, if one is of a very gross, physical, and insensitive nature and demeanor, their network of spiritual pathways never has been very active or of great dimension. These are the people that one would call very physical versus very spiritual even in common terms. They like to eat pork, red meat, hunt animals, involve themselves in sports, and other activities that are very much sensational or sense-stimulating.

This is not to say that these are evil, unkind, or bad people. A great many of them are wonderful, friendly, generous, kind people. You may see them at church every Sunday, maybe teaching Sunday school. Another way to say this is that they are functioning very much in the "outer" world, and these positive activities may be the better side of good behavior in an effort to simply be a better person. This is all well and good, but in the Bible it is said that we would be doing the same type of works that Jesus had been doing and even greater. I don't see many people doing these works and this is one of the reasons why.

You have to be REALLY active spiritually to be able to manifest these things in your life, and those spiritual channels must be huge and channeling immense amounts of spiritual energy. I mention this to illustrate the differences that I am trying to present. Most people have no idea of how great they can become when they practice proper spiritual techniques and turn that ego into a servant rather than a master...a slippery slope indeed. Lots of effort, training, and time are involved, not to mention dedication. There is a quantum difference between the two worlds, spiritual and physical. You must bridge it to be successful. Most people who do alternative healing are somewhere in between a life of pure physicality and pure spirituality.

Now we have a veritable Pandora's Box to have fun with. To help with understanding, it is helpful to remember that the mind, thoughts, and emotions are all resident objects of the spiritual realms. They are not physical in the least, although they feel that way; but that can be explained too. Now back to Pandora and her Box. Thoughts provide definition, shape, or meaning for energy so it can be useful. You might think of a spear or an arrow. In and of itself, it can do nothing but lie there and look like a spear or arrow. It is not dangerous in the least.

Emotions are the force which, when applied to thoughts, give them force. In the above examples, it might provide the force to (not to be confused with power which requires authority) either hurl these objects, which might now be classified as weapons, at some target or withhold some action. Thoughts provide little or no action, only definition. Emotions on the other hand provide the force (hopefully, power) to move, hurl, lift, expand, contract, etc. that which has already been provided with form and definition.

The most important part of this whole discussion is to understand that the mind and the energetic or spiritual structures are all on the same dimension, much the same as our physical bodies are on the same dimension as would be a spear or arrow. That is why the effects of these same-dimension things are so profound and effective. The third element (after thought and emotion) is will, or intention, that directs thoughts and emotions, without which there is no reason for any of it.

To return to the gist of how the Interference Principle functions, there is something that I call the "Oneness Principle". This is because of the unifying role this concept plays. Ultimately, all is one, including you and me. When we engage in negative or harmful behaviors, of whatever degree, it shrinks our spiritual bodies and channels thereby reducing the creation gradient principle.

The life-giving and creative flow of life, which is supposed to course through our being, is reduced or strangled. Not only that, but the chakras and the channels related to these areas, and any places of weakness of the "target" person, are where these negative energies attach. This is an example of like attracts like.

It is helpful to remember that thoughts and emotions are things, with one having definition and the other having mass on their own dimension. They can easily separate from the energy body of the sender and fly like the proverbial spear or arrow into the other person. Then, what goes around comes around. Through the Oneness Principle, the sender gets it too. If the sender was not harmonious with it, they would not have had possession of it in the first place.

When one uses these energetic weapons damage is done, whether intentional or not - and saying that you didn't know it was damaging or that it was an accident makes no difference - it was still done. Like a child breaking a window with an errant baseball, accident or not, it still was done. These energetic influences find their mark regardless of the sender's intention and clog, disturb, drain, tear, or otherwise interfere with the circulation of the Life Energy in both sender and receiver.

These influences are being channeled into the incarnated soul (soul body) and cause disturbances both directly and indirectly to the energy body and tissue function. Can you imagine a blood vessel performing properly with a big knife stuck through it? The blood vessel just won't work properly in that condition.

The mind is so much more powerful than one might imagine. It creates connection, which Pranic Healing practitioners call "cords." These are like tubes that extend from one person to another and transmit life energy, or prana, in whatever manner the person doing the thinking or intending, happens to have going on within them at the time.

Usually the cords are of a draining nature, so it's sort of like having leaks in your system, that literally suck the life out of you. The reasons many are unaware of this include that the "leaks" are so small that you don't notice them and most people don't know about this energetic mechanism. Of course, there are ways to prevent and remedy these problems; or I wouldn't have brought them up.

Since the tissues receive the Life energy that differentiates them from simply being a piece of meat, disturbances in the energy flow into the incarnated soul body will result in disturbed function on the physical level or dimension. This is a law that cannot be broken, because it is one of the Laws of Creation that feeds and sustains all living beings. It is responsible for growth, healing, function, and regulation. Usually, the disease processes that issue forth from these disturbances are the ones for which conventional "medical science" cannot find the cause or cure.

The reason for this is that science is required to avoid areas of interest and investigation that are not physical or chemical or offend the traditions established by history - not to mention the financial interests. Whenever conventional methods cannot determine or substantially relieve a condition, look to the non-physical for the answer. More often than not, you'll find it there if you search properly.

The tissues must be fed on two dimensions or there will be disease. I hope that you can see that there are two distinctly different ways that the flow of Life, or Prana, through the individual can be compromised. Also, there is not an easily defined line of demarcation between them but a somewhat substantial amount of overlap.

It must not be forgotten that some disease processes reside entirely on the non-physical; but since the mind is incapable of distinguishing between energetically-based and physically-based pain and disability, what may be assumed to be physical may actually be entirely energetic.

HOW EMOTIONS ARE INVOLVED IN HEALTH AND DISEASE

Emotions are a force or power depending on how, or if, they are qualified with authority of some kind. Authority refers to an influence derived from a responsible source. Force lacks responsibility. Also, this depends on whether they are focused on destruction, construction, prevention, disturbance, or resolution. For those of you who actually have a working knowledge of the difference between power and force, they are being used in this section interchangeably for the purpose of simplicity of writing and convenience.

In the usage of these two words, this is true for most of the content of this book; but there is a big difference between the two, that difference being: force can be mindless movement of energy regardless of intent and result. Power has, as its guiding influence intelligence, ethical purpose, and hopefully wisdom and love. The negative of these are also true and effective. Of course, this is only an abbreviated definition, but it helps provide clarity. Another way of saying this is that force does what it does simply because it can and power does what it does because it ought to, or has a reason to.

Many emotions fall into the destructive category simply because the individual involved is not aware of what is happening. I don't want anyone to feel guilty when reading this, even if they have perpetrated great harm on someone else intentionally. What I would rather see is that they use the power of emotion, guided by proper thought, to resolve and heal themselves and those that they have harmed.

This does not necessarily mean that there has to be reconciliation, but that they learn to stop doing the harm, reorganize themselves to a higher purpose, and learn to provide healing to those they have harmed. Pranic Healing and Reiki are good examples of suitable techniques that may be effective in circumstances such as this.

As stated above emotions are the "motive" or driving force in both the damage and the repair of the energy body and the trickle-down effect it has into the physical. Again, it is the Law.

Certain emotional states result in specific types of problems. These relationships are based on a number of different factors. Certain chakras manage a specific range of energies. The specific chakra can be determined by the emotional influence processed by that chakra. This not only gives emotional influences an identity but a destination, like attracts like. This is known as the Law of Similars. The same goes for certain meridians. Also, in accordance with the meridians, the Eastern system of five elements is involved and each has certain tissues that are managed by them.

There is also a commonly used system of four elements. This is more commonly used in the West. The Western system of four elements: Fire, Air, Earth, and Water are more useful for describing how things are created, or constructed. This has more to do with some of the methods of European metaphysical thought. The Eastern system of five elements is more concerned with how things function. It's a little similar to the subjects of Anatomy and Physiology. Anatomy is the "what is it and what does it do" compared with Physiology which is "how does it do what it does and why". In this text, our main area of interest is in the how and why.

The energetic (Chinese) element system is comprised of five elements that encompass the characteristics of the principal energies and combine to enable, or explain why, how our systems to work the way they do. Again, the Western system uses a four element system of Air, Earth, Fire, and Water to represent basically the same things; but the four element system of the West is inadequate for human functional purposes.

The Eastern system combines the fire and air in its fire element, and adds wood and metal for a total of five elements. This completes a five-pointed star configuration which empowers a higher complexity that adds greater control to the system. The different combination incorporated by the Eastern system, better accounts for living things and controlling factors. The Western four element system may be more applicable to astrology, which has other influences to explain things such as houses, signs, and planets, but not so much for growth and control factors. Please see the diagram below.

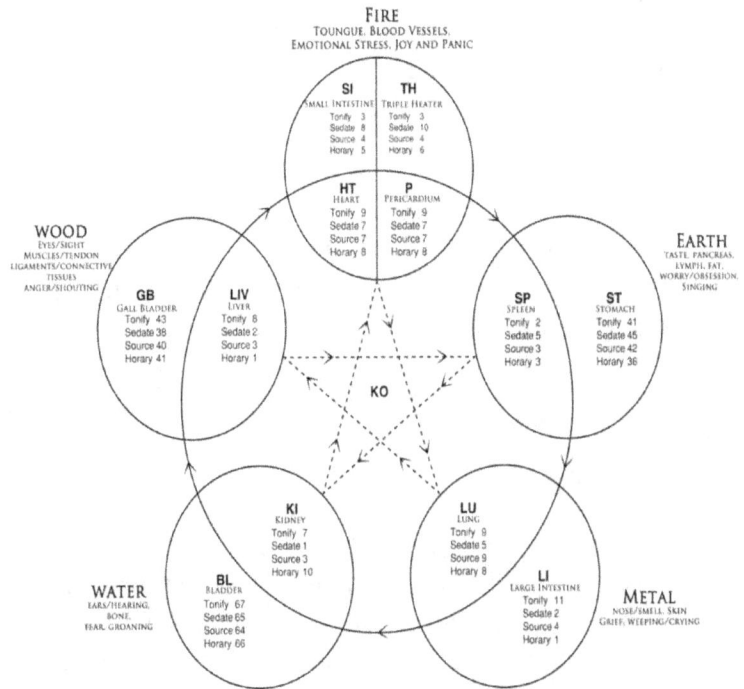

The fire element, which includes the small intestine, triple heater, heart, and pericardium meridians, responds to excess emotions. The associated tissues are the blood vessels and tongue. When these are out of balance it means that a person has been over-emotional or has some emotional influence upsetting their internal balance. Stress is one of the more common examples. These people have a tendency to experience episodes of joy, panic, and possibly, hysteria. This element has a tendency to influence what goes into the body. This affects the heart, wrists, digestion, neck, and internal balance. Fibromyalgia and carpal tunnel syndrome are good examples of common problems related to the fire element and emotions. Of course, there are a number of additional problems as well.

The earth element has a strong influence on the pancreas via the stomach and spleen meridians. The associated tissues are the lips, lymph, and fat. The emotions associated with this element are worry and obsession. Again, there is some influence in terms of what goes into the body and how it is digested, absorbed, and processed. Diseases typical for this element and its meridians are diabetes (especially type II), anorexia nervosa, irritable bowel syndrome, Crohn's disease, menstrual cramps and most forms of dysmenorrhea, ovarian cysts, premenstrual syndrome, and endometriosis.

The metal element encompasses the lung and large intestine meridians. The associated tissues are the skin, thyroid, body hair, and mucus. The emotion associated with the disturbance of these meridians is grief. Just as grief buries itself in one's heart, this element may have the influence of burying things in the system which should not be there. This could be the loss of a loved one, a pet, some object of affection, or even having left the mother's womb unwillingly. Typically, asthma may result, plus toxic disorders due to the nature of these meridians and the organs they serve. These have to do with elimination of toxins and wastes to the outside of the body.

Another symptom is pain at the base of the thumb (thenar pain in the first carpometacarpal joint area) which is difficult to differentiate from arthritis and may be combined with arthritis. Also this may explain why people who are really clean in terms of toxins have clear skin and beautiful hair.

The water element is involved with the ears and hearing. The tissues associated with this are bone, head hair, and saliva. In case you are wondering why one of the tissues could possibly be bone, consider that it is the blood (about 97% water; blood is produced by bone) that is the medium by which the minerals for bone, mainly calcium, and phosphorus, are transported. These are transported, including the hormones, calcitonin, and parathyroid hormone which control bone density, by the blood both to and from the bone. Hair is no different. The operative emotion is fear.

In the Western system especially, emotion is symbolized by water. The kidney and bladder meridians are of the water element. They both manage watery functions and are involved in elimination of wastes and toxins, to the outside of the body. This is a logical follow-up to the metal element that may have been involved with the removal or retention of toxins which could be part of an unhealthy process. Some organs remove toxins from a tissue, such as the blood tissue; but that does not get those toxins out of the body.

The Wood element is more for growth and structure in some respects. It involves the liver and gall bladder meridians with the related tissues/organs which are muscle, tendon, ligament, and nails. It also involves eyesight. Anger is its pathologic emotion. Interestingly, when you find a person who is chronically angry, they often have liver or gall bladder problems. In alcoholism, the liver is compromised; and there is often a pronounced behavior of anger, especially when drinking or stressed.

The operative mechanism in the development of disease is the altering of the flow of Life's Energy through these meridians. The chakras are no different in terms of alteration and contamination due to the same influences as the meridians experience.

The word "chakra" is a Sanskrit word for "spinning wheel". Unlike the meridians, which are the counterpart to the circulatory system (the blood vascular and lymphatic systems) the chakras are the counterpart to the organ system. They each have different sizes, colors, locations, and functions...just like the organs. They also become contaminated, or toxic, just like the organs.

The chakras and meridians serve as "magnetic targets" for emotional influences, both positive and negative, because of the Law of Similars; and this is where thought-forms and emotional influences can become lodged. They not only clog and block the functionality of the chakras but actually alter and "poison" the energy coming and going through the chakras. This can pervert the energies of chakras and cause some very unusual things to occur within the individual suffering from these problems.

The chakras can develop holes and cracks which alter their function. An example is cracks in the solar plexus chakra resulting in compulsive eating disorder. Into these openings and weaknesses can lodge, or even enter therein, various thoughts and emotions that then attach to the psyche, changing emotional and thought patterns unconsciously. The person doesn't even know it's happening to them. What I am trying to say is that they know it's happening, but they don't know why. It seems to be out of their control, or at least almost so. The reason for this is that the control mechanisms of the individual have been altered by a foreign influence.

In the Bible, the removal of these influences is called the "casting out of demons." Grand Master Choa Kok Sui, the founder of Pranic Healing, likens them to "psychic cockroaches". What he is trying to say is that they aren't such a big deal; they just make a big mess. Pick them out and throw them away like the "bug" that they really are.

Detailed functions of the chakras of both their energetic properties and physical influences are taken from the writings of Master Choa Kok Sui is as follows.

There are many, many chakras, but the older and most common system utilized only 7 chakras. The newer system introduced by Grand Master Choa Kok Sui utilizes 12 major chakras. This includes the aforementioned seven but adds others including some "minor" chakras. Of course, these chakras have always been there; but as the Teachings evolve, the system becomes more expanded. I do not use a numbering system, but a naming system. The numbering system has its variances among different users and can lead to confusion, particularly when attempting to learn another system with more components.

Chakras are very much like our physical organs. They become "toxic" when impurities become lodged in them. These impurities, of course, are energetic in nature and come in all forms – from attached elemental beings (beings, often called nature spirits, who have the majority of their existence within a certain realm of creation and are not physically visible and are often not very evolved, although some are) to thought-forms. The character of the impurity will determine which chakra will be affected and how.

At this point a listing of the chakras, their functions and the organs they influence, is in order. Usually, their location is fairly indicative of the organs they influence due to their proximity.

Basic Chakra – located at the back of the pelvis at the base of the spine in the region of the coccyx. It controls and energizes the bones, muscles, spine, blood, and both cellular and general growth, body heat, plus it affects the heart and sex organs. It is the center of self-survival, or self-preservation.

Sex Chakra – located at the pubis in the front of the pelvis. It controls and energizes the genitals, urinary bladder and urethra, the legs to some extent, and the throat and head (as the energy naturally rises). It is the lower creative center whose energy is utilized by the higher centers in creation and intelligence.

Meng mein Chakra – located at the small of the back just above the pelvis and behind the navel. It controls and energizes the kidneys, adrenal glands, and regulates blood pressure. It acts as a pumping station moving energy up the back channels of the spine.

Navel Chakra – located at the navel. It controls and energizes the small and large intestines, the appendix, the speed of giving birth, and general vitality. It helps in the circulation of prana within the acupuncture meridians.

Spleen Chakra – located just inside the lowest portion of the rib cage on the left side. It controls and energizes the spleen, affects the pranic and general vitality of the body, and affects the quality of the blood and the immune system. It is closely related to the navel chakra and serves to energize a number of the other chakras.

Solar Plexus Chakra – located just below the inverted "V" that the rib cage forms at the front of the chest a little lower than the heart. It controls and energizes the diaphragm, liver, pancreas, stomach, to a substantial degree the small and large intestines, adrenal glands, heart, and lungs. It energizes a number of other chakras and is the center for the lower will and is easily disturbed by negative emotions.

Heart Chakra – located in the middle of the sternum immediately in front of the heart. The heart is actually located in the center of the chest, and the apex (point) is the only portion of the physical heart that is left of center. It controls and energizes the physical heart and conditions the blood on energetic levels. It is the center of higher, or refined, emotions. It balances the lower will with love and higher emotions in a very direct manner.

Throat Chakra - Located in the throat about midway between the jaw and the sternum. It covers the area of the larynx (Adams apple). It controls and energizes the throat, larynx (voice box), trachea, thyroid gland, parathyroid glands, lymphatic system, and it all affects the sex chakra. It has a strong relationship with intelligence.

Ajna Chakra (also called the Brow Chakra) – located between the eyebrows. It controls and energizes the pituitary gland and the entire body. It controls all of the major chakras and the endocrine system, and it affects the vital organs. This chakra is the center of the higher or abstract mind and is also the center for the higher will or directive function.

Forehead Chakra (also called the third eye) – located at the center of the forehead. It controls and energizes the pineal gland and the nervous system. This chakra is the center of the lower buddhic or cosmic consciousness.

Crown Chakra – located at the crown of the head. It is the entry point of the divine energy. It controls and energizes the brain and the pineal gland. It is the center of higher buddhic or cosmic consciousness.

Twelfth Chakra – located about one foot above the head. In Christianity it is known as the Pentecostal Fire. (See Acts 2:3) It may be helpful to recall that the energy body is larger than the physical body therefore some parts of the energy body may be located beyond the skin. This is the seat of the incarnated soul.

HOW THE ENERGETIC SYSTEM OF HEALING WORKS

Probably the best way to describe how the energetic system of healing works is to describe it in two ways. This is because there are two principles by which energetic healing operate. The reason for this is that there is an interdimensional transition that the energies concerned must make, and there is a "state of being transition" that must be accomplished.

First, the interdimensional transition, or shift, is one of a "creative" nature. What this means is that even from the physical perspective, it is one of creation. Actually it is of manifestation, but the creation perspective is appropriate in many ways. For it to be wholly creative is possible but much more unusual in our conscious experience. This "creative" system is one of facilitating a down-flow of energies for the purpose of supporting something already physically manifest which is already living, or having life. Also, in this perspective, it is presumed that a healing, repair, or alteration process is the desired end result.

The process is one of accessing the appropriate energies from the appropriate sources and applying them in the appropriate manner to the appropriate areas of interest. You may notice that there is a lot of appropriateness involved here. If these areas of interest in appropriateness are not managed properly, the desired result may not be achieved; or there may be other problems that arise that could have been avoided.

One of the first areas of appropriateness is the source of the energy that is being used for the process at hand. There is any number of sources for this energy. One form is animal sacrifice...not acceptable for many reasons such as karmic reactions, etc. Another is taking that energy from another person, plant, or animal...also, not particularly a proper thing to do. You know karma and the like; it's something like being a thief. You may draw the energy from within yourself; and while this is acceptable, it is not wise.

If you do this, you are temporarily depleting yourself, at the very least. Also when people do this, they have an unconscious tendency to draw energy from others; and this has a negative effect on those from whom they have unconsciously drawn this energy. They have then incurred a spiritual debt to them. You can beg the energy from other beings that are generous to a fault, such as trees, friends, and animals with which you share a connection that would bear such a transaction. Again, it is a debt. You can ask God for it directly; but if that were to actually occur in real life, you would be incinerated on the spot due to the need for intermediaries for the purpose of "stepping down" the energy as transformers do with electricity.

The best way is to be connected consciously with real-life qualified teachers who actually do the kind of work that you are proposing to do and can do it much better than you can. Often we call these great beings "masters". This is much different than some who have achieved the level of Reiki master or a master plumber. That is only a level of recognition within a generalized energetic transference practice or trade and does not convey what the title "master" really means. In Western society, the title Master is very little understood as to it what it takes to become one of these great beings with that title.

The most appropriate manner in which to obtain the energies with which to apply healing is to get it from the Great Teaching and Healing Masters and their assistants. This is what they do. In principle, there can be no receiver without a giver. Likewise, there can be no giver without a receiver. According to this line of logic, there can be no destination without a source or vice versa. A simpler way of explaining it is that of a stick; it must have two ends. For energy to flow along this pathway, which the provider of healing must be part of, either as the channel or standby controller, there must be a gradient...a concentration gradient. These by universal law flow from areas of more to areas of less.

There is an entire company of higher beings that got where they are by teaching and providing a greater abundance of blessings for those who have not yet developed the ability to manage that much Prana, chi, life force, or whatever you want to call it. It is similar to being in a stream but wanting to position yourself in the location where the flow is the greatest so you have more to work with. Also, the energy, chi, Prana, etc. that is channeled through them, is usually purified by them assuring a higher quality of service to yourself and your client.

These Great Beings are the "step-down" stations for the energy that comes from God for the purposes of whatever your intention is. They funnel the energy "down" into you at your request, and you access it from within your own system. What is happening in reality is that you are using some of your own energy and a lot of theirs, which they are replacing faster than you are receiving it. The proper manner in which to access this is found in the book, Advanced Pranic Healing, through chakra utilization. But, there is an additional benefit - that when you do this properly, you end up with more energy than when you started, and have generated positive karma, and feel wonderful yourself.

In short, upon your request, the Great Beings get the Prana, or energy, from God and pass it down a descending line of beings greater than yourself (which advances their evolution to an even greater degree so they can do even more service) to you. It's a concentration gradient thing, scientifically speaking. It's holistic and helps build the "greater community" and includes you in it. That covers the first two areas of appropriateness in a summary form.

Remember that when it comes to these types of practices, it is no different than another type of flow. A river flows along its course; and if it passes through areas of natural purity, it remains pure; but if it passes through areas of impurity, it carries with it those impurities with which it has come into contact. This is why some practitioners are more suitable for some clientele than others. Impurities also will flow along/down a concentration gradient. Everything does.

The third case of appropriateness deals with the application of the energies in an appropriate manner. This means to use the right type of energy. Remember, there are not only the energies of Fire, Earth, Metal, Water, and Wood, but there are different frequencies that are commonly expressed and visualized as colors. You should be well-educated in these things before you get in very deeply or attempt to treat serious conditions. If this situation presents itself, call for the assistance of a qualified healer; or use the simple methods you do have at your disposal and invoke for help from the Higher Beings. They will do the fine tuning and even alter what you're doing if you mess up badly enough...but be sincere in your asking for help.

What all this means is that a LOT is possible with the right intentions, knowledge, and training. Don't skimp on any of them. If you are even reading this book, I am assuming that your intentions are to be a great healer...or even aspire to become a Master. Well then, do it! And never back down from your goals!

The amount of energy introduced into the recipient is also required to be appropriate. Harm can be done if the recipient is given too much energy or if it is done improperly. This is where proper training comes in. The very sick, aged, and very young are the most susceptible to problems arising from receiving too much energy.

Balance is also important. One of the principle concepts in healing is balance. What this means is that a major goal is to achieve balance within the entire being of the recipient as much as possible with the means at hand. Scanning, a method of "feeling" or sensing the part being evaluated, or worked with, is a crucially important skill to have developed. This helps provide a guide so you know what to do or not do in your attempts to aid your fellow beings.

The use of an improper energy can be very destructive. Remember, your goal is healing; and if your goal isn't healing or positive uses, but simply attempting to learn the basis of personal power, your efforts will backfire as surely as the sun rises in the morning. Remember the concentration gradient. The energy must go somewhere; and if you are hoarding it for personal power, the flow will most likely back up and be destructive to you in ways that you never would have imagined. Now we can move on to appropriate places.

Where the energy is applied is very important. Not only does the affected part need to be properly energized in the proper manner with the proper type of energy at the proper frequency, but remember we are doing this right and not simply messing around with what we think we know but what we actually do know. There are some areas of the body that would simply respond in a minimal manner when energized improperly, or with the wrong energies. There are other parts that might prove destructive if the "healing" energies were to be applied there. It's something like a recipe for supper. You use the right ingredients, or it gets messed up. There are some recipes that can be abused and others that cannot. Energetic healing is no different.

As the energy is introduced into the physical system, it must be assimilated, or absorbed. This requires certain factors to be present. First factor is a favorable "concentration" gradient, so the energy will be able to flow. Now that the flow has been established, it must be able to enter into the recipient. This requires receptivity on their part, both mentally and emotionally. If this is not present, the activity takes on the character of coercion. Permission must be granted, whether it is assumed or requested; it must be there.

FACTORS WHICH AFFECT A PERSON'S SUSCEPTIBILITY TO PHYSICALLY-BASED DISEASE

To begin with, a positive outlook on life is essential, and after that, a healthy diet and regular exercise. Of course, these are related to the mental and psychic. When outlook, diet, and exercise are suffering, there is a negative "trickle down" effect. These can result in obesity, physical weakness, decreased mental functioning, poor self-image, and various other undesirable traits. As the general state of the person declines, they are more prone to accidents, poor judgment, infectious diseases, and a downgrading of the related energetic components of their entire system. The spiritual cord that feeds them their life energy decreases in size, and they don't have as much to work with on any level. Their access to their God-given resources of Life is diminished to the degree that their connection with the Source of Life is reduced.

Stress can be one of the most significant factors. While stress is a very general term, in this case, it is meant as emotional or lifestyle stress. Most emotional stress affects the energetic components of the being, especially since emotions are on the same dimension as the energy structures. But that is not where the damage stops. It affects the central nervous system and glandular systems, including the endocrine system. This has a profound effect on the physical system in many ways. Digestion is altered and along with it the entire digestive tract including the large intestine. The heart and blood vascular system is altered in function; and this reflects through altered function of the kidneys, the most homeostatic organ of the body. Many people do not realize that the kidneys and the heart work in constant unison in regulating blood pressure.

When a person is stressed, often they are distracted. This can lead to poor judgment and accidents. Of course, this opens up a list of possibilities far too long to address in this text, so I'll leave you to your imagination. Be careful not to dwell on these things too long though. What you think about is what you attract into your life experience.

In short, most of the things that affect a person's susceptibility to physically-based disease are actually energy-based. While the cause often is energetic, the result is physical…and that's when we notice it. So often, we have no idea what the actual cause was when we find ourselves with an affliction. This indirect approach to accidents and disease is all too often unrecognized by our health professionals and distorted by the tales and folk lore that so many rely upon for understanding what is happening to them and why. Another step down that slippery slope of folklore is depending on it for the curative actions found there. A major confusing factor is that so often the folklore way is often correct, or at least, partially so.

HOW WHAT YOU EAT, WEAR, AND HOW YOU LIVE AFFECTS YOUR PERSON

Now this could be a "can of worms" quite easily. We have so many customs and familial ways of doing things, especially eating. Often, someone is diagnosed with a "hereditary" disorder, usually by asking if others in the family have had the same condition. Often, it isn't hereditary, but familial...a learned, or habitual activity that results in disease. This usually involves one's dietary habits. Diabetes is a favorite disease to become encumbered with this influence.

Some of this can also be attributed to the latest penchant of medical science which is genetics! Often when the conventional medical system cannot ascribe the etiology of a disease to something infective or chemical, they turn to genetics. Sure, genetics has its problems, but a lot of things are being pinned on genetic problems that simply don't belong there. Also, genetics can change upon appropriate stimulus to that part of the system (for more information, refer to the study of epigenetics). Remember that all of the cells all contain identical DNA.

What you wear is also a factor. The fabric can affect you not only because of the fabric itself, but also the color. The fabric has electrical, thermal, and chemical characteristics that can, and do, affect you. This ranges from allergies to heat stroke. The color has its influence too. Color denotes frequencies of energy; and these frequencies attract, repel, and alter the energies coming and going to and from the body. They affect the functioning of the energetic systems of the body and the perceptions and reactions of other people.

At the top of the "bad" list are the synthetic fabrics. Some are worse than others. At the top of the "good" list are the fabrics made of natural fibers such as cotton, wool, linen, etc. Not only can this affect people but pets as well. Some time ago, I moved into a house that had carpets made of something my dog was allergic to. He would constantly be scratching and biting at the area in his lower back and above his tail. Much of his hair fell out and he was miserable. We got another dog, and the same happened to her. We thought fleas might be the problem, as they were quite attracted to the dogs' compromised state of health.

When we moved them to another house where there was no carpet or synthetic material, the itching stopped and their hair grew back. The same is true for humans with their clothing. The example of the dogs was included simply as an example, although somewhat extreme. I'm sure that some of you reading this will be able to say quite honestly that this not an extreme example and that the same fate has befallen fellow humans with similar results.

Eating is one of the biggest problems Americans have. We are constantly lied to and intentionally confused as to what is good food and what is not. We have developed into the one of the most obese cultures on Earth. All this is with the blessing of our wonderful government. Many people trust the government to be the watchdog for our dietary well-being. Not so! Sure, sometimes they do things that keep the most unscrupulous of commercial interests from selling us things that we should not eat, but so often what they approve is almost as bad, and sometimes worse.

The key here is two-fold: education and proper supply. We need education so we actually know what is good for us and what is not. Our society has become so busy with unimportant activities and trying to be self-important and impressing others that we all too often succumb to slick advertising that tells us that we should drink this or eat that. Of course, beautiful bodies that are selling us this bill of goods don't eat that stuff. It's just another commercial lie. The schools don't educate the children in such a way that they can tell what is OK to eat and what is not, especially by example with their government-advised "school lunches". Anybody want a double helping of Thursday medley surprise? I cringe at the thought.

On the supply side of things, how does one actually find and purchase proper food in this country? It is not such an easy task if you want to do a really good job. If you want to do a halfway decent job of it when you go to the supermarket, shop along the outer isle of the store. That's where all the food that's still alive is. All the dead, canned, dried, and nutritionally scary foods are in the middle of the store. Sure, the veggies are grown with herbicides and pesticides in mineral-depleted soil, but at least it's still alive. The dairy products are fractionalized and adulterated, but they still have some of their original nutritional properties.

Of course, the best is fresh, organic, raw food that is not in the form of leftovers. The soil in this country is mineral deficient, and often we need to supplement our diets with the minerals that are lacking in the soil.

Malnutrition is a habit, custom, tradition, and a disease! Obesity is a result of malnutrition! This is not starvation, but a perversion of starvation. Too much of some things and not enough of others constitutes malnutrition. Look around you. What do you see in terms of other people's health and weight problems? Do you see health? Even in the collegiate environment, there is much evidence of what I speak.

FACTORS WHICH AFFECT A PERSON'S SUSCEPTIBILITY TO ENERGY-BASED DISEASE

Reactivity in general. Reactivity has the special quality of placing the one reacting in a position of being controlled by that to which he/she is reacting, pure and simple. This is a very direct relationship between the two components of this type of activity. Many people do not realize that they have choices regarding the means by which they manage incoming influences. Often, people comply, resist, or somehow attempt to change that influence. The idea here is to choose between two polar opposites; reaction or response.

Reaction implies the receiver is being controlled, either consciously or subconsciously, and the source of the influence is the controlling factor. When engaging in a response, the receiver is in control. This does not mean to imply one should not be receptive to what is being given them, even if the intent of the giver is to impose or control. Without reception of the influence it cannot be dealt with in a positive manner, only avoided, which may be the best strategy.

Using certain martial arts as an example, a response offers options that might be compared with the technique of using an opponent's momentum, strength, or weight to their disadvantage. It's sort of like the old saying: If given lemons, make lemonade. A key component to having this type of strategy available is to be aware of the options as they present themselves in the first place. Fear and non-thinking severely hamper one's ability to employ useful strategies when imposed upon by outside forces.

Being "disconnected" from the here and now also disconnects one from being aware and effective on very basic levels. Often, one can be heard saying "If only I had known that at the time...and it was right there in front of me." This is an example of a lack of perception or some level of unawareness, both of which are the absence of being fully present, which cannot really take place if one does not exercise receptivity on some practical level.

Social factors often are closely related to internal factors (there is considerable overlap between these two) and are usually those factors that are normally seen in person's relations with or reactions to others. This can take the form of depression, fear, pride, greed, and most of any of the other social disgraces we either inflict on others or accept upon ourselves. Often they result in the development of the "internal factors" immediately following this subtopic.

One example that comes to mind that fits well into this category is that of carpal tunnel syndrome. This is a condition that has been attributed to overuse of the hands and wrists while improper bodily posture and ergonomics are practiced. Historically, this is definitely inaccurate, although a few cases are sure to exist. Instead of the median nerve being interfered with as convention insists, the pericardium meridian traverses the same part of the upper extremity in very precise fashion. This particular meridian has four names that come to mind: pericardium, circulation-sex, heart governing vessel, and heart constrictor meridian. The path of the inner portion of this meridian must be seen and understood to understand the reason for these many names; but for our purposes here with carpal tunnel syndrome, we will use the name "heart governing vessel".

In this instance it is the feeling of being obligated against ones' will to perform some sort of task or activity. In a phrase, "doing something that one's heart is not in" is descriptive of the character of the pathologic emotion involved. When this pathologic activity takes place, the energies of this meridian are stifled and the hand and wrist become painful to use. After a lengthy period of disuse, the muscles at the base of the thumb and those directly across from it, the opponens muscle group, atrophy from non-use.

It is interesting that a physiologically-based test, electromyography is used to "scientifically" establish the diagnosis. If this were an actual inflammatory, over-crowding condition, as is purported by the medical authorities, why would they not use an anatomically-based test such as an MRI? The most logical reason I can come up with is that the MRI would not show anything as being pathologic, so a test is used that will give some sort of reading that is useful to the purposes of the surgical community and the insurance industry.

More on carpal tunnel syndrome and its relief can be found in the Treatment Manual, available separately. To pique your interest; just let it be mentioned that acupuncture uses needles to puncture the skin therapeutically, so what is happening on a practical, physical level when the scalpel enters the skin and the sutures are applied with a suture needle? An unintentional acupuncture treatment is what takes place without the surgeon being aware that this is what is happening. This is what causes the assumed success of the surgery.

Internal factors are things such as misgivings, self-doubt, confusion, disbelief, and pain (either physically-based or energetically-based pain). These are usually the after-effects of outer events that we have either internalized or self-created out of our varying levels of confusion about how life really works...or the way we wished it works. Due to the myriad of different emotions and conceptions/misconceptions in which we engage, the results of these types of internal misappropriation of our energies can cause almost any outer problem to become evident. This is where psychiatrists and psychologists feed.

Social, religious, familial, and unhealthy "entertainment" influences are usually at work here, with the victim reacting to such input, when it should simply be discarded – or better yet, not engaged in, in the first place. Usually it is the "adoption" of someone else's problem, then becomes the recipient's problem, then can devolve to become a "can of worms" that is nearly impossible to sort out. It is much simpler to discard the whole mess, forget the past with which it was all associated, and begin an entirely new belief system that is healthy.

It is in this area of activity that the psychologist/psychiatrist can be useful – not just nursing the problem along. I would encourage anyone with these types of problems to study the work of Tony Robbins, the originator of the "success coach" movement and "self-help" author. In the absence of a formal education, and likewise the "academic tunnel vision" that it engenders, through observation and insight, Mr. Robbins became one of the leaders in mental/emotional health world-wide. He has put together systems of practice that have the potential of refocusing one's inner attributes to very effective levels.

Reactivity factors (guilt, fear, shame, anger, emotional stress). These are the five pathological emotional patterns described by traditional Chinese philosophy. They are each associated with a specific element that includes both a yin and yang meridian, specific tissues, specific organs, senses, etc.

Clinically, I have found this as a very applicable base-line philosophy on which to anchor my inquiry regarding the inner mechanisms by which a particular problem is manifest in a patient. The details for each of these factors and their related five elements will be presented later on in this text. When examining this area of philosophy, a great deal of latitude must be exercised, all the while remaining focused on the implications of the particular case at hand. Interpretation is the key rather than strict, by the book, logic.

Environmental factors include chemical pollutants in any part of the environment that can be brought into the body's system such as food, drink, air pollutants, medicines, and the like.

Genetic factors. I'm sure we have all been misinformed about genetic influences on our physical bodies. So-called "science", not to demean actual, true science, says in their eternal partial wisdom, that behavior is purely habitual or non-physical. Sometimes it is cast into that scientific nether-world called "research." The simplest way to debunk this assertion is to ask any farmer who raises animals. Of course, farmers who farm entirely grains, and have no animals, would likely agree with their animal-raising brethren on this issue. If you actually do ask a farmer if behavior is an inherited trait, invariably, the answer will be "Of course it is." Keep it simple. The farmers are very practical and don't use advanced mathematics with which to confuse themselves. They use simple observation...generations and generations of it, which is the foundation of true science.

When someone is very expressive and reactive, we might think of this person as being Italian. We call it ethnicity, but it is actually genetic. A person of Italian descent, but born and reared in Chicago, may exhibit this behavior but the Italian genetics are there, hence their behavior.

Spiritual factors can include the misapplication of spiritual healing practices, kundalini syndrome (a condition of mishandled energy/power derived from advanced meditative practices or even physical injury to specific energy-sensitive areas of the body), surgically cut but not reattached energy channels in the body, emotional insults that are taken to heart, and other things that have no physical basis of origin.

These spiritual, or energetic, influences disrupt or divert vital currents of Life within the system which results in imbalances that become evident as disease-like symptoms; but they have no physically verifiable origin. Usually, it is the behavior of organs and tissues that becomes disturbed not the physical matter itself that can be biopsied and examined under a microscope.

Physical injury factors are a particularly confusing area of concern. When a physical injury occurs, say, one in which a person falls or is struck by an object, the impact has two basic components, one is physical, the other energetic. One is a collision of matter against matter, the other is a pathologic vortex introduced into the flow of Life energies as they pass through that part of the body. This usually takes place where an acupuncture meridian passes through the tissues. After the physical injury heals, proper function is not completely restored, leaving both patient and physician confused as to why a portion of the problem persists.

Usually this shows itself as the inability to move properly in terms of range of motion, pain with or without movement, and eventually atrophy of the tissues involved. To resolve such a problem, it first must be determined whether the basic nature of the problem is physical or energetic. Usually in these circumstances, the physical aspect of this is already taken care of by the healing ability of the body and maybe a physician; so simply jumping to the conclusion that the problem is of energetic nature is usually accurate. Simply restoring the flow of energy through the tissues by applying micro-current in the correct polarity along the energy channel, usually a meridian, will resolve the problem immediately. Sometimes it is a simple matter of applying appropriate energy to an acupuncture point, usually in the approximate vicinity of the problem, is all that is necessary.

Effort-induced factors. This might be better explained by relating an event that took place in my clinic. One day, a strong, healthy 28 year-old man entered my office complaining of shoulder pain. I examined his shoulder and found no physical problem whatsoever. Usually people such as this do not have shoulder injuries unless they have been heavily involved in sports, which he had not. Upon very specific questioning, it was revealed that he had tried to move a very large, heavy object by using his shoulder to push it.

The particular detail that was both difficult to arrive at and bring out into the open diagnostically was that, while he pushed with all his might, he did not move the object whatsoever. All he did was apply effort...as opposed to force. In this case, force being a physically applied activity and effort being a pathologically intense intention activity, injury is possible. The difference here is that force would injure the physical components, but effort would have the ability to injure the energetic components. As soon as some energy was applied to the large intestine meridian point on his shoulder, the problem instantly resolved.

It is important to note that a thorough physical evaluation was performed previous to the application of electrical micro-current. If micro-current is applied before the proper understandings are arrived at, the addition of that restorative influence may well confuse the clinical picture by masking an actual physically-based injury, thereby exposing the patient to a greater likelihood of serious re-injury. It was the force of intention that injured the meridian due to the degree of his intention, that of pushing with his shoulder; and it was not his musculoskeletal anatomy that sustained the injury.

Surgically-induced factors are simply the cutting and not reattaching of the energetic components of the patient. This is often a hit-or-miss affair due to the restorative capability of the individual patient, the spiritual conductivity, intention of the surgeon, and the connecting or blocking characteristics of the tissues involved. Really, it's a wait and see situation for the most part. The most evident of these would be what is sometimes referred to as a "toxic scar".

These scars are often painful, tender, reddened, and generally "unhappy" tissues. In cases such as these, the energetic capability and conductivity of the tissues has been interrupted and has not been able to adapt. In these types of cases, micro-current applied in both polarities is applied in every conceivable fashion across the scar to. The other major variant of the surgically-induced group of problems is that the energy channel is cut, does not reattach and re-establish proper flow, and the "downstream" portion of the meridian is underserved and underfed. This "starves" the tissues of Life energy, and they misbehave and atrophy as would any previously fertile land would in a drought.

Additionally, this major lack of flow or blockage causes a backlash effect throughout the sheng/ko (constructive and destructive influences respectively) cycles of the yin/yang balance and elemental systems. This elemental balance system is created in such a way so as to produce a dynamic balance of the energies of life.

THE EXPECTED RESULTS OF AN ENERGY-BASED DISEASE WITH A PHYSICALLY-BASED TREATMENT

When physically-based treatment is rendered for an energy-based condition, often there is a response of one result on another result, without the causative aspect being addressed whatsoever. In other words a symptom is being treated, not the cause, and the treatment is the result of the practitioner's mistaking the dimension on which the problem actually resides, hence one result applied to another. Symptoms are a result of a disease. These two "results" are the symptoms on one hand and the body itself on the other. The physical body is the physical manifestation, or result, of the energies of Creation.

The physically-based treatment is likewise of the same nature. The problem is quite clear that the cause is not being addressed. If the actual cause is left unaddressed, it is perfectly logical that the condition will remain unchanged with only temporary modifications in its symptomatic expressions.

As an example, consider that there is a body of water that has some disturbing force acting upon it in a regular, predictable manner. This would provide a certain type of turbulence. The shape of this turbulence we call "symptoms" due to its difference to what the character of the water would be if this disturbing force were not present, and it were left to its own natural expression.

If we add to this disturbing force another disturbing force, for instance one that counteracts the first disturbing force to which we assign the identity of a certain "disease", it may appear that such "disease" is "healed". Due to the fact that the original disturbing force has not been changed or altered in any meaningful manner, the actual disease persists; and the appearance of healing may become evident. This is a typical example of trying to rectify one effect with another.

Basically, what we have here is an "identity crisis" of sorts. The identity of the original disturbance may have been noted, although not accurately identified as to its actual nature or even the dimension on which it resides. Physical logic says to do this and that, but the necessary considerations are incomplete.

The result of attempting to resolve energy-based disease processes via physically-based treatment modalities is nearly always ineffective due to their existing on different dimensions and in different places within the creation continuum.

If the causative energetic disturbance is not corrected, the disease will continue to persist and return and return. Energy provides behavioral information to the tissues; so it stands to reason if a tissue, like a person, misbehaves long enough, they will degenerate beyond useful purpose and be separated from the rest of the population of tissues or simply fall by the wayside. Diseased tissues that result from these processes of "misbehavior," are more prone to infection and cancer. They often result in the destruction of the entire organism. This can be directly interpreted as leading to death of the person or long term misery and discomfort.

Energetic disease being treated on the same dimension on which it resides, and in a perfect world with perfect understanding of energy-based disease, will rectify the actual energetic entity that was at the root of the problem to begin with, usually an out of balance emotion directed by a poorly defined and placed thought.

PART FOUR

THE BASIC RELATIONSHIPS OF THE SUBTLE (ENERGETIC) PARTS OF THE PERSON TO THE PHYSICAL

These relationships are both direct and parallel. This equates to the phrase "direct and proximate", but "proximate" would be inaccurate as it pertains to something that is nearby, not occupying the same physical space. The physical and subtle, or energetic, are within each other, with the "parallel" aspect meaning that they are on adjoining dimensions of Creation. One mimics the other, but not exactly, which also supports the term "parallel". An easy to provide example would be considering the mind and the brain. When considered by physically-oriented persons, they see no real difference. As an example, consider the two words "ground" and "earth".

These have many interpretations and uses but are often considered the same by some, but there exist many differences. In the example of mind/brain, the similarities are few when adequately understood. An easy to understand example would be to consider the difference between a computer and the operator with the brain as the computer and the mind as the person operating the computer. They are more "associated" than "connected". The same is true of the body and the being that inhabits the body.

The computer gets old and is replaced, the operator simply obtains another computer; and the body gets old, dies, and gets replaced, and the being obtains another body (reincarnation) with the mind continuing with the being, since it is likewise energetic in nature. In the last analysis, even the physical is energy-based but of such a low frequency that it is too gross to transcend the differences that exist between the "human/body" and the "soul/mind" except in very few instances.

To enter into greater and functional detail regarding the energetic and physical, certain similarities exist in shape, color, size, and on functional levels.

COMPARATIVE OVERVIEW OF THE BASIC PHYSICAL AND SPIRITUAL SYSTEMS

With a little thought it is not difficult to understand that nothing physical can exist without a basis for that existence. Since everything physical is made up of molecules, which are made up of atoms which are made up of positive, negative, and neutral electrical charges, the understanding that even physical matter actually is energy is evident.

What is left to understand is the organization of the energy into physical objects. While this is quite easily recognized scientifically, what we have not recognized very well is how the purely energetic and grossly physical relate.

Plainly put, everything physical has an energetic pattern on which it depends for its existence; otherwise, it would disintegrate. It has to have a "creation/created" reason for being what it is. Everything physical shares this system. Every cell, tissue, organ, organ system, and organism has, at its core, a mirror-like energetic "double" upon which the physical portion of this dual reality is based. When we try to discern this as an absolute rule, it works; but when we try to apply an exact "picture reversal" sort of interpretation, it's not quite so clear. This is likely due to our flawed understanding of the actual spectrum physical creation occupies.

Every physical organ, tissue, function, or any other part of the human "system" has its spiritual counterpart, basically, in both form and function. This, in plain words, means that they have a similar appearance and activity.

This can be directly illustrated by the following comparative list:

Physical	Spiritual
Organ	Chakra
Blood vessel	Acupuncture meridian
Nerve	Nadi
3 layers of Tissue	3 layers of the aura

Organs compare closely with chakras in a number of ways. Organs are in different locations, of different colors, different sizes, and process substances differently according to their individual identity. Chakras are in different locations, of different colors, different sizes, and process energy differently according to their individual identity. There are approximately seven major/vital organs and seven major/vital chakras. Of course, there are many more organs; and likewise, there are many more chakras. Specific organs function with specific chakras in the support and function of specific organ activities, and often the chakras share the same name as the organ such as the heart chakra.

The chakras also function along the same lines emotionally as the organs they pair with. An example is the sex chakra which is functionally involved with both the functioning of the sexual organs and sexual emotion, along with the solar plexus chakra. The autonomic nervous system controls, nearly in its entirety, the physiologic functioning of the sex organs.

Blood vessels compare with acupuncture meridians in both flow and function. Blood vessels are of many sizes and are well distributed and located in nearly all parts of the body. They transport life-giving substances and nourishment to all tissues and carry away waste for disposal. There are about five different things that are moved about by the blood vascular system. These include transporting food, water, heat, waste, and gases. Acupuncture meridians do much the same on energetic levels by transporting the energies of the five-element system of Chinese philosophy of fire which includes air, metal, water, earth, and wood. The elements relate directly to specific tissues and organs of the physical body and establish a harmonic balance between the physical and energetic/spiritual halves of ourselves.

Nadi, which is a Sanskrit word that directly translates to "psychic nerve", carries information from place to place within the energy body quite the same as the physical nerves do in the physical body. They seem to be of primary importance when doing yoga or other forms of self-evolution and development beyond "normal" levels. It is interesting to note that the greatest concentration of major nadis in the energy body is along the spinal cord and in the brain. The same is true of the physical nervous system. Actually the physical body and spiritual body are superimposed upon one another in a very direct manner. The nadis come in a variety of styles. Some of them are purely energetic channels; some combine with muscles, blood vessels, lymphatic vessels, and nerves.

Nadis are found in two major types: subtle and gross. The subtle nadis include the channels of mind (manas) and the channels of feeling the "self" or "being" (chitta) that which fills the mind. The "yoga" nadis are included in this category, and often information is difficult to find regarding them, as details about them are often kept confidential by the traditions that maintain this type of knowledge. Additionally, there is the fact that this knowledge is absolutely useless to anyone other than a practitioner of very advanced yoga.

The staff and serpents of the medical caduceus represent several of these channels. In fact, the so-called "medical caduceus" is actually the Staff of Hermes who is known in Greek mythology as the messenger of the gods. Hermes is also known as the god of science, commerce, eloquence, cunning, and the guide of departed souls to Hades – a lot of import referred to in the use of this style of caduceus. The more accurate symbol for the medical profession would be the staff of Asclepius, an ancient Greek physician who became known as the god of healing. His staff is represented with a single serpent wound around it.

Nadis manage foundational issues such as regulating and regulation of levels of consciousness and foundational energy balancing functions of the energetic system of the individual, in a phrase, frequency management and quality control. Nadis carry an energy called "prana", which is a Sanskrit word meaning the "breath of life"; and in Christian terminology, it means the "Holy Spirit."

The gross nadis are channels of subtle energy that have the character of chords, vessels, or tubes. These are included in the concept of acupuncture meridians, nerves, muscles, and the streams of the cardiovascular system such as arteries, veins, and the lymphatic system.

You may notice the rather marked difference of the spiritual compared to the physical nature of the two types of nadis. The "physical" nadis are the energy character of the physical organ in which they are found. The subtle nadis function on a higher order, or level of the individual.

The aura has three basic layers which are, from outside to inside, causal, mental, and emotional. There are many interpretations of how these are described, especially regarding the innermost layer. It is sometimes called the inner aura, astral layer, or other things. The physical body, from outside to inside, goes from skin to muscle to bone. Likewise, the physical developed from three embryonic "germ" layers that are, from outer to inner, ectoderm, mesoderm, and endoderm. You may have noticed a predominance of 3's here. These "trinities" are not by accident.

WHICH PART OF THE PERSON IS IN CHARGE AND WHY

This can be a tricky question, because it depends on one's point of view...even before the consideration of subjectivity and objectivity becomes involved. From a Creation to manifestation perspective, things naturally progress from an idea, to a plan, to a concept model, to a working model, to a mass produced model. This indicates that there is some intelligence involved in this from the beginning regardless of one's personal opinion. This is an exercise in impersonal functionality not personal belief which may be dictated by many varying factors – one more obvious and or practical than the other. To support this idea, it is noteworthy that science and spirituality actually support one another and religion and spirituality often don't. Never mistake a belief in something for the thing itself.

    The basis of the matter is that the flow of creation goes from the Creator to the created, meaning from the subtle toward the gross in both density and down the scale of frequencies. In the finest of analyses, this indicates that it is the subtle which is in charge; for without it, the gross would not exist. On the other hand, the lower nature of the individual has the capacity of interfering with the mechanisms of the higher nature of the individual and very often does exactly that.

    The manifestation of disease then becomes the natural outworking of the energetic or creation part of the individual who is in a corrupt, but natural, state. It is here that belief (subjectivity) and the thing believed in or not believed in (the thing itself, regardless of belief) comes into friction. We can identify that difference of opinion as that which impedes one's ability to seek out appropriate health care management applicable to their specific condition, beginning with differentiating between the physically-based and energetically-based types of disorders.

WHY THE PHYSICAL COMPONENT CONFORMS TO THE SUBTLE

Years ago, in the science classes I attended, the explanation of how the various complexities of the human body were developed was based on "cell differentiation" and such vagueness of concept. After many science classes through the doctoral level, never did I hear of a better explanation; as the topic was quite ignored. The geneticists of today probably have a much more elaborate way of explaining these processes but complexity does not make a basic concept any truer if it is wrong to begin with.

Nothing happens by accident, simply due to the fact that anything that happens must have some causative force and defining character to it for it to take place at all. The development of an entire human body arises from simply the genetic components of its beginning, the ovum and sperm, each of which contributes a haploid number of chromosomes to the now nearly complete cell. These then replicate to produce the normal diploid set of chromosomes of a normal, complete, cell as is found in the human body. So how is this "intent" or causative impetus managed?

Who or what is directing this physical show? After all, it takes place with great precision and predictability. How is it, that even the smaller arteries are developed exactly where they should be? How does the thyroid gland know where its borders should be with such fantastic regularity? Actually it goes along the same lines as the universe. The universe is extremely well-ordered on an incomprehensibly immense scale as is the working of the inner functioning of a single cell. There is an energetic plan and intention already in place. It is to this energetic, or spiritual, form or framework that the lower density, or physical atoms and molecules, cling and create the form you see before you in the mirror or another person or animal.

How can one imagine that the extremely immense complexity and detail of the physical and biological world is not even more immensely complex and detailed in the energy world? It is by necessity due to the "direct and parallel" nature of our universe and world(s). It can be said that without a course down which to flow, the stream would not exist.

Referring back to the comparison of the physical components and the physical and energetic bodies, even these must have a well-defined and well-detailed plan of action. This is provided by a higher spiritual function that has been termed the "physical permanent seed" which, like a seed that is planted in a garden, is embedded in the heart chakra.

Grand Master Choa Kok Sui says in his book, The Spiritual Essence of Man: "The physical permanent seed is located in the heart chakra – Chesed (in Kabbalah), and the physical heart. The physical permanent seed is also called the 'life seed,' since it gives life to the physical body. From the higher soul, soul life energy is infused into the physical permanent seed from where it is distributed into the different parts of the physical body, making the body whole and integrated. It also gives the physical body the ability to absorb prana. Once the soul life energy is withdrawn from the physical permanent seed, the body dies."

There also exist emotional and mental permanent seeds that serve similar purposes in their own special areas of definition and function. For those who question the unusual levels of intelligence displayed by some individuals that seem inconsistent with other aspects of who they appear to be, the development and effectiveness of these "seeds" may provide a clue. In a sentence, brain function and intelligence are not necessarily directly proportional.

WHY AND HOW THE SUBTLE (ENERGETIC) COMPONENT BECOMES DISEASED

The basic concept in this topic is that of inappropriate misplaced power resulting in corruption of an otherwise appropriate and healthy process. I don't think anyone will argue that emotions can be powerful influences in our lives, but it is often not understood or realized that this power is not without effect. Since we are so distracted with the physical side of life, we forget what destruction emotion may create.

Taking into account that accurate information is necessary for any proper communication to take place between multiple components of a complex system, it is not difficult to understand that if such communication is corrupted, the messages, or instructions, delivered result in activities not originally intended.

The two primary systems being referred to are the acupuncture meridian system and the tissues themselves. On either side of this duality of function are thoughts and emotions which provide the input and the tissues providing the expression of the original intention. The energies carried by the acupuncture meridians direct and dictate the behavior of the tissues.

This behavior is not to be confused with the function of the tissues. As an example, a muscle contracts – which is the function of that tissue and organ; but the manner in which it contracts, or the reasons for its contraction, constitute its behavior. To be more graphic, it is the difference between a person receiving an object as a gift, or having earned it, or simply stealing it. The person still gets the object, but by different means. It's the character of the action not the action itself.

In human physiology, a classic example would be the passageways of the lungs; when they are behaving properly, they dilate and constrict according to the physiologic needs of the person. When this person has the condition we call asthma, their respiratory passageways constrict and dilate improperly, or more accurately stated, inappropriately. The reason for this is an energetic corruption of the lung meridian.

This corrupting influence is a "pathologic" emotion, most often the emotion of grief or intense loss. Grieving is a natural process; but when engaged in for too long a period, or too intensely, it becomes a pathologic status in one's life rather than the temporary influence it would normally be. It is counteracted by the dynamic auto-regulating character of the sheng and ko cycles of the five elements and yin and yang energies described in Chinese philosophy. This is a self-correcting system; but if impacted in too great a degree, or for too long a period of time, it becomes affected over the long term which we then term a "disease" such as asthma. The cause remains and is not rectified until an outside influence, such as acupuncture, Auriculotherapy, or micro-current corrective therapy, or some other therapy, rebalances the system and returns it to its natural order.

With the corrupting influence in place, the aforementioned pathologic emotion, the tissues receive "bad" information and, therefore, begin behaving badly.

Due to the fact that the acupuncture meridians are one of the principal providers of Life Energies, including what we call Prana, Chi, Qi, Holy Spirit, or others, these fundamental energies provide basic and crucial support to the physical tissues on a cellular level. When these problems continue over a long period of time, usually many years, as in Crohn's disease, the tissues gradually become markedly debilitated.

To further use Crohn's disease as an example, this disease can be reversed in short order with few residual problems; but if it persists for many years, the process of rehabilitating the tissues on a cellular level becomes necessary. This normally takes years of careful diet and lots of energetic healing care. The two principal modalities that come to mind would be pranic healing and Auriculotherapy using both phases 2 and 3 of the ear (in the advanced levels of Auriculotherapy, the reflex points move to other regions of the ear depending on the age of the condition, and these are called phases) . Other modalities can be selected, but these two are the most focused that I am aware of.

PART FIVE

THE COMPONENT CHARACTER OF THE SUBTLE PART OF THE PERSON:

THE FIVE CHINESE ELEMENTS

Different cultures have different philosophies that have on their fundamental, baseline, foundational level something we call "elements". The European system has four elements, being Air, Earth, Fire, and Water. These are fine for certain uses, particularly in the occult traditions having to do with metaphysics. In the healing practices, the system that seems to be more appropriate and works better is the five element system of Earth, Metal, Water, Wood, and Air/Fire (Air and Fire being combined to form the single element of Fire). Each of these elements have within it two acupuncture meridians, one yin and one yang; and Fire consists of four meridians, two yin and two yang.

It should be noted that these elements describe the character of the energy of which they are composed. It is sort of like the visible light spectrum being made up of different, distinct colors; the elemental energies are also quite separate characters of energy, vibration, frequency, and color. When one observes a rainbow, they can clearly see the different colors distinctly; and where the colors are adjacent to one another, their joining is neither crisp nor gradual. It is a distinct demarcation between the two frequencies, or colors, with but little combining.

This provides an easily discernible and visual example of a "quantum" difference between the two colors in question. It is either one or the other with little, if any, being a combination of the two. The five elements of the Chinese system of elements are much like this. The situation of the Fire and Air being combined can be likened to the fact that their energies are not as quantum-defined as would make them different on a practical level. It is like the difference between pink and light red with not enough difference to make it practical to separate them from one another. However the meridians associated with them are quite separate.

The sheng and ko cycles represent the relationships that exist amongst the five elements and provide a dynamic balance for the whole, which would then require a substantial impact for the result we call "disease" to take place. This topic will be taken up in greater detail in following parts of this text.

PRANA, CHI, QI, THE GREAT SPIRIT, AND THE HOLY SPIRIT

For many of the civilizations throughout history and even at the present time, there have been different names for "That" which makes life exist here on planet Earth. We refer to God as being the Supreme Being beyond either description or understanding. Radiating outward, or downward, from this Source of Life is where the various names come into play.

As this "downward flow" takes place, manifestation on all levels is enabled. It's sort of the opposite of water evaporating and more like steam (the atomic state of water – invisible, and not wet) cooling to become water vapor (the particle, or droplet state of water – visible and moist), condensing to become liquid water (wet and much more palpable), to becoming ice (cold, solid, and brittle). As you can readily see, the only difference between these four states of water is the temperature and pressure of them. There are definite states of structure in terms of the state of matter in which water is being observed or experienced.

The spiritual world is much like the various states of water, being more or less subtle, depending on the vibratory rate. The greater the energy and higher the frequency, the less "solid" it is. As in the rainbow, these frequencies occupy certain locations within the scheme of things. The rainbow "contains" specific colors in a specific position within its structure; and then the overall structure, or shape of the rainbow, is likewise predetermined by its natural or inherent nature. What this means is that energy, when in the manifestation process, travels down certain, natural, predetermined pathways toward a predictable destination.

In the human system these pathways are more complex and varied but follow the same sense of order as everything else in Creation. Now that we have brought to the fore that there is something with which to contain and direct these energies, what flows down and through these defined pathways is of primary importance.

For the sake of simplicity, I will refer to this energy that has so many names as simply "prana". Prana is something like electricity, as it can take many forms and be used for nearly anything. Like electricity, it is purely energy. Prana comes to us in many forms such as air prana, plant prana, earth prana, and solar prana – each with its own unique character. Hopefully this will help make the Chinese five element system a little easier to understand, especially to the Westerner.

Probably the easiest to observe is air prana. When gazing into a clear blue sky with unfocused eyes, there may appear small, mobile "blips" of silvery light. It's almost like seeing a fish in the water on a sunny day dash near the surface and then swim quickly back into deeper water. Another attempt at describing air prana is observing the punctuation mark, the comma, as an alive and mobile thing with many of them swarming about before one's gaze.

What are actually being observed is "vitality globules" given this name in the early 20th century by C.W. Leadbeater. These have the form of a child's "spinning top", an old-fashioned conical toy that was pointed at the bottom, larger at the top; and when spun, it would stand on its point and dance around until its rotation became too slow to support its upright position. These vitality globules have within them a spiral structure in which the whole thing has an inner and outer motion which is continually moving.

When these are seen in a very condensed form, they appear to be a beam of light. They are visible to the mind but not the brain; therefore, it is not the eyes that see them but the minds' eye. For those familiar with more scientific terminology, the vitality globules are visualized by means of perception (mind, awareness) rather than sensation (brain, nerves, eyes, etc.) Hence, all is not as physical as one might have guessed.

Through meditation, prayer, and other practices, the prana is brought into the system and directed as desired, providing one has the education or knowledge with which to manage this. In the shortest of explanations, it is by intention that energy is directed. Where your attention and intention are directed, is where the energy from your system goes...period. The only way to alter this law of life is to invoke for help from more powerful and cooperative Beings than yourself to manage how and where these energies are directed.

Everything is energy. Physical objects, bodies, and matter are simply solidified, manifested energy. This is not just mysticism; it is science, specifically quantum physics. It requires a great deal of energy to manifest changes in the physical body. It is much easier to use solidified energy for solidified bodies, (physical treatments for physical problems). The use of energy for healing physical problems does work however there are not many healers in the world who are capable of channelling sufficient amounts of energy to cause these changes in the physical plane in a short amount of time. It takes time and tremendous amounts of energy to manifest something physically without using a physical catalyst. For example: it is far easier to grow an apple from an apple tree than it is to manifest an apple with no tree.

The use of energetic healing modalities, such as the use of directing vitality globules toward a problem, works far more effectively on energy-based conditions; but it also works on the physically-based conditions as well, just not as quickly or intensely. There are several factors that limit the energy treatment on the physical condition; these are the amount of energy being applied, the ability of the recipient to receive and assimilate the energy, and the severity of the condition – which determines how much energy will be required. This whole thing works better in one direction than the other, hands down.

YIN, YANG, THE FIVE ELEMENTS, AND THEIR NATURE

Yin-yang is a conceptual framework which was used for observing and analyzing the material world in ancient China. In the I Ching, or, The Book of Changes, the most ancient of the Chinese classics, it is said that "Yin and yang reflect all the forms and characteristics existing in the universe." "Yin and yang are the laws of heaven and earth, the great framework of everything, the parents of change, the root and beginning of life and death..." Basically yin and yang provide the duality that makes all manifestation possible.

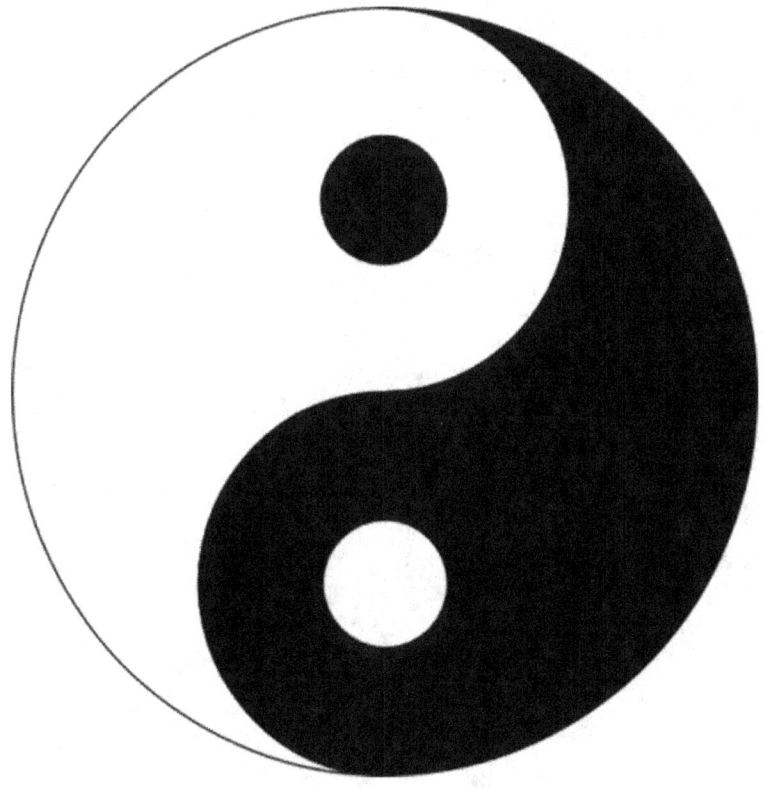

They may represent two separate phenomena with opposing natures as well as different and opposite aspects within the same phenomenon. Probably the most classic examples of yin and yang are represented by water and fire. While this system of definition, being ultimately pervasive throughout our universe represents opposites, it also represents balance. This balance is on such a fundamental basis, that it is nearly incomprehensible to the human mind. It is absolutely basic and foundational.

To further complicate one's attempts at understanding something so foundational, these two opposing forces of nature are found one within the other and are inseparable. They create the gradient down which creation manifests and create the current of everything becoming what it is. The yin yang symbol is depicted as a circle made up of two curved forms, one black and one white, with a central dot of the other in each, a white spot within the black and a black spot within the white.

This represents the dynamic balance found within all creation that both promote its existence and growth yet limit and control this growth so order may prevail. When disease is present, this sense of order has been violated such that balance between these two primal forces is upset beyond its innate capacity to rebalance itself. According to Chinese philosophy, all disease can be classified as being of either yin or yang nature. Yin and yang are both opposite and constantly and continually interacting and interpenetrating one another right down to the levels of the subatomic particles studied in quantum physics.

The five elements refer to five categories in the natural world. The theory of the five elements holds that all phenomena in the universe correspond in nature either to wood, fire, earth, metal, or water; and that these are in a state of constant change. This theory, or conceptualization, was first formed in China around 221 B.C. Historically it derives from observations of the natural world made in early times in that wood, fire, earth, metal, and water were considered to be the five indispensible materials for the maintenance of life and production, as well as representing five important states that initiated normal changes in the natural world. A quote from A Collection of Ancient Works is "Food relies on water and fire. Production relies on metal and wood. Earth gives birth to everything." Therefore, in early times it was understood that these five elements represented certain, specific things in life.

These five elements represent five different characters of energy and activity. The character of wood is to grow and flourish; the character of fire is to be hot and flare up; the character of earth is to give birth to all things; the character of metal is to descend and be clear, and the character of water is to be cold and to flow downwards.

HOW THE FIVE ELEMENTS INTERACT TO CREATE BALANCE AND IMBALANCE

Also in Chinese lore is the law of movement of the five elements. How these five elements relate to and affect one another is of vital importance in both the maintenance of health and the restoration of health in the case of disease. The understanding of these movements and influences is crucial to understanding the basic inner balances of the human system of energy structure. These movements, described by their character of behavior, are termed: interpromoting, interacting, overacting, counteracting, and mutual interaction between mother and son. Promoting implies promoting growth. Wood promotes fire; fire promotes metal (as in the fires of the refining processes of extracting metal from ore); metal promotes water, and water promotes wood.

Acting, as used in this section, means the bringing under control, or restraint. To illustrate the importance of restraint and control, consider the humble single-celled mold micro-organism. If a single mold cell were given optimum nutrition and environment without any restraint whatsoever, it would double in population, with one cell becoming two, two becoming four, four becoming eight, and so on, with the entire population doubling with each reproductive cycle. Rather than simply pose the question of how much mold would be produced in a 30 day period, the answer is given...in 30 days of perfectly promoted growth, the Earth would be covered over its entire surface with a layer about thirty feet deep. Now, whether you believe this or not is immaterial; but the concept that controls and limiting factors are essential and foundationally important cannot be dismissed. It is an absolutely crucial requirement.

Always consider what the words used to describe specific things or activities actually mean. This includes the parts of the words under consideration. Examples include: promote, meaning to initiate something in a forward direction or manner, and the term "interaction" meaning "an action that is taking place involving two or more components." Without actually reading into the text the actual "mechanical" parts of the definitions, so often the strength of the intended message is lost and its true import left unrealized. Become a philosopher to enough of an extent that a clear understanding of what is being communicated is actually understood.

The pattern of interpromoting (the term "interpromoting" in this context is the equivalent of the term "promoting", so the word promoting will be used) contains fire promotes earth, earth promotes metal, metal promotes water, water promotes wood, and wood promotes fire. An easy way to visualize this is that the more wood you put on a fire, the larger the fire becomes. This constitutes the sheng, or building, or expansion, cycle of elements. Rather than attempt to detail the names of the elements and the rationale behind their names compared to their positions, such rhetoric will serve no useful purpose at this juncture.

The ko cycle is the inhibiting, or contraction, cycle of the elements. These relationships function as interacting and overacting influences and are represented by wood against earth, earth against water, water against fire, fire against metal, and metal against wood.

A third set of relationships between these characters of energy we term "elements" exist as the counteracting relationships. In this instance, the influence is directly counter to the sheng cycle; and if the sheng cycle were represented as a clockwise diagram, the counteracting influences would be going in a counter clockwise direction, skipping the first element encountered in its backward direction and acting on the next one encountered. Therefore, the counteracting relationships are fire counteracts water, water counteracts earth, earth counteracts wood, wood counteracts metal, and metal counteracts fire.

The above represents a composite and a complex of activities that can be considered a trinity of influences that maintains a dynamic equilibrium of the energies that constitute the organization of the denser levels of the energy body.

THE RESULT OF IMBALANCE OF THE ELEMENTS

When considering the manifestation of disease in the most reasonable order of development, from Creation to the created, it is vitally important to understand the basic components of the system. In this part, we are concerned with fundamental energetic identities being at odds with one another.

This comprises a foundational corruption, or disturbance, in how the grosser levels of the inner being operate. These imbalances, for whatever reason they are present, throw the energetic dynamic equilibrium out of balance beyond its capacity for self-correction. This imbalance, usually initiated by emotional trauma, physical trauma, inappropriate diet, poison, or energetic impact from attack, energetic body damage, karma, or other unfortunate experiences suffered by the individual can lead to all sorts of misery. The key to unravelling these cases is to have an all-encompassing conceptual awareness and knowledge so that nothing significant is missed in the evaluation of the situation.

An example of this can be illustrated by the case of a woman who had 28 surgical procedures on her right lower extremity after a fall in the bathtub. After a very careful and detailed inquiry as to the exact nature of the fall, what part of the body was impacted, the nature of the pain, etc., it was determined that she had indeed injured her right gall bladder meridian, the imbalance of which resulted in non-neurologically mediated pain, which the conventional medical community pursued with surgical and chemical philosophy and method. This is a classic example of an energetically-based condition mistaken for a physically-based injury. She was eventually crippled on a practical level by the conventional efforts at symptomatic resolution. The question may arise as to exactly what her physical injuries were…who knows…but likely just bruising and maybe a sprain, which would resolve by themselves if left alone and not reinjured.

Another classic is what is referred to in Auriculotherapy as a "toxic scar." In this instance, the energetic channels have been severed; and when the ensuing scar tissue develops, a non-conductive barrier is created. This is where micro-current is very useful in re-establishing conductivity to the area in question.

In the case of emotional impact, the pathologic emotions are disruptive to a degree sufficient to throw the dynamic balance of the elemental and meridian system out of equilibrium such that it cannot recover on its own.

Having a firm grasp of the principles involved in this work is the most practical means of being effective in these healing practices. In summary, this means understanding the principles of frequency, the power of emotion, the conduction of information, and the double nature of the human being.

The intent of this work is to simplify and render practical for the interested individual or practitioner a whole spectrum of healing ability that was heretofore perceived as very complex and mystifying, although in principle this is not necessarily so. This is not to say I do not respect the traditional Chinese medical system or its philosophy, because I really do. It's just too cumbersome for the advocate whose interests are not directed that intensely toward it and a more manageable system utilizing these principles is therefore in order.

THE PRIMARY PATHOLOGIC EMOTIONS AND THEIR RELATIONSHIP TO DISEASE

There are many, many different emotions, so many in fact that it is both impractical and useless to attempt to catalogue them. Instead, it is helpful to know that they can be grouped into basic characters of energetic impact. These generally defined emotions serve a practical purpose in the organization of understanding the mechanisms of what we term "psychosomatic disease." Furthermore, the more intricate details of these emotions may serve to identify the portion of a body area served by an element or meridian in terms of what disease the victim may experience.

Examples for the stomach meridian include anorexia nervosa, Crohn's disease, irritable bowel syndrome, menstrual cramps, and others. While all of these problems are the result of worry or obsession, or some combination of both, it is the finer detail and identity of the emotion (its signature frequency) that determines the organ or tissue along the course of the meridian that will respond to the corrupted message being transmitted. It is very much like a radio station transmitting a specific frequency and the receiver (household radio), or in this case the organ and its matching frequency, responding to it. This can be considered as sort of a "lock and key" arrangement, whereby they are different from one another but also fit together.

The inherent disharmony results in aberrant expression of the energies being communicated by the affected system.

These disharmonies are as follows:

Element: Fire. Emotion: Emotional stress. Meridians affected: Triple warmer, heart, pericardium, and small intestine. Tissue affected: Vessel – blood and lymph. Examples of resultant diseases: Carpal tunnel syndrome, cardiac problems, and fibromyalgia.

Element: Earth. Emotions: Worry and obsession. Meridians affected: Stomach and spleen. Tissue affected: Muscle. Examples of resultant diseases: Menstrual cramps, diabetes, premenstrual syndrome, all sorts of dysmenorrhea, anorexia nervosa, irritable bowel syndrome, and diarrhea.

Element: Metal. Emotions: Grief, sadness, guilt, and melancholy. Meridians affected: Lung and large intestine. Tissue affected: Skin and hair. Example of resultant diseases: Asthma.

Element: Water. Emotions: Fear and fright. Meridians affected: Kidney and bladder. Tissue affected: Bone. Examples of resultant diseases: Blood in urine without physical cause, exquisite pain parallel to the spine, and pain in the sole of the foot.

Element: Wood. Emotion: Anger. Meridians affected: Liver and gall bladder. Tissue affected: Tendon. Examples of resultant diseases: Gall bladder problems and migraine headaches.

The diseases listed above do not constitute a complete list, but these are the most common and obvious general examples.

Sheng Ko Cycle with Element and Meridian Details

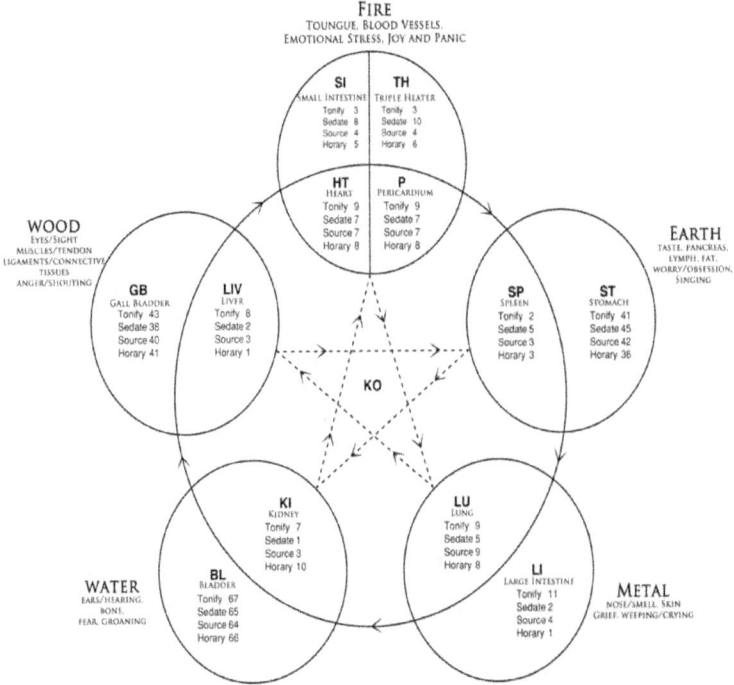

PART SIX

THE "CHALLENGE SYSTEM" OF DISCOVERY

(The mechanical basis of EET therapy)

In order to present this material in a more coherent form, likely some minor review is in order. The energy body anatomy has within it many points of activity. These have been termed chakras, acupuncture meridians, and nadis to name some of the principal ones. Meridians deliver to the tissues behavioral information. Chakras process energy.

Acupuncture points are "access points" by which the characteristics of the meridian being treated can be influenced or modified. Both acupuncture points and chakras have a spiral or rotational character, which is further illustrated by the fact that the acupuncture points along a given meridian tend to cycle in order through the five elements of the Chinese system of energy philosophy. The chakras also have their associated element with the five-element system, and the chakras and acupuncture points can be likened to the others with having similar characteristics of being both control and access facilitators.

The main difference is that they are of different sizes. They form an ascending/descending sized energy structure, the acupuncture points being of various sizes and the chakras also being of various sizes. Chakras are generally larger than acupuncture points with the exception of micro chakras.

Considering that the practitioner's hand contains within it the energetic component that is providing the "challenge" part of the mechanics of challenging a point/meridian for purposes of evaluation, then the acupuncture point/meridian would constitute the "challenged" part of these mechanics.

This obvious difference in the size as demonstrated by the chakras can be understood as major chakras, such as the heart or solar plexus chakras; the minor chakras, such as the spleen or liver chakras; the mini chakras, such as the chakras of the soles of the feet or palms of the hands; and the micro chakras, such as the chakras in the tips of the fingers found on the finger pads.

These micro chakras found on the pads of the fingertips provide the practitioner with the faculty of communicating with an acupuncture point or meridian on its own level and in the appropriate energy amplitude for effective information or influence transference to take place. Simply stated, the micro chakras and the acupuncture points are of similar size and power; therefore, they can interact with one another easily and effectively. This form of communication represents the question being presented to the patient's system. This is how the patient's system is employed for the purpose of "dousing" or obtaining direct or comparative information as used by some practitioners of Applied Kinesiology and similar arts.

When used as a determinant in discovering the appropriate meridian or acupuncture point for treating a health issue, a neutral state of mind and emotion are essential; otherwise, the communication process will be corrupted. To effectively neutralize this corruptive tendency, some level of detachment by the practitioner is necessary combined with a sense of "curiosity." This helps immensely to clear up practitioners' confusing the evaluation process with their own misgivings.

This "neutral" method of communication is foundational to accurate and effective communication with the patient's system. The issue at the beginning of the evaluation is the discovery of whether the problem being addressed is of physical origin or energetic/emotional origin. Of course, do not neglect the characteristics and details of the history which provide very salient data from the beginning of the case.

In this type of general communication with the patient's system in a basic evaluation, no questions are being posed to any part of the patient's system other than "Is this of benefit or not of benefit?" The result is interpreted in the most general sense as to whether the pain on palpation of the alarm point for the meridian in question is relieved by the specific challenge.

In general summary, and to help clarify this procedure at this point, it goes like this. A person comes in to have their problem addressed. On taking the history, it is suspected that their problem may be of an energetic nature. The type of problem may be generally "suspected" by knowing which organ or tissue is involved. Thus guided the practitioner gently but firmly palpates the alarm point of the meridian being evaluated. Then, the practitioner simply touches points along the meridian (preferably tonification or sedation points, or those in the area of complaint) while again palpating the alarm point. Points that relieve the pain of the alarm point are then considered for treatment. If a particular point relieves the pain found at the alarm point, that meridian is further confirmed as being considered for treatment.

If there is no pain at the alarm point for a given meridian, then that meridian is not as strong a candidate for treatment.

It is extremely important to understand the relative factors involved in the meridian system that involve the sheng and ko cycles. Sometimes a meridian is the "victim" of another meridian, and therefore, is part of the symptom rather than the cause. In such cases, the meridian causing the trouble is not the one under treatment; and the exercise is simply one of chasing symptoms rather than addressing causative issues. Almost always, the actual cause is one of emotional imbalance or trauma, physical insult or injury that has an unaddressed energetic component, or some other undetermined but energy-based issue.

WHAT DO I NEED TO BE ABLE TO DO THIS ADEQUATELY?

First is an adequate working knowledge of the energy and physical systems of the individual and how they relate to one another. Second is the ability to keep things both logical and simple conceptually and in practice, as confusion and complication court failure. Third is one must not interfere with the patient's energy system, either by introducing confusion from their own emotional or intellectual influence or disturbing the patient's status by inappropriate input into the equation.

In short, keep your hands, emotions, preconceived notions, and any non-confirmed attempts at treatment away from the patient (and out mind) until you have a reasonably accurate idea of what the patient's problem actually is, what you are doing, and why. While this whole system is quite safe, it can be confounded and confused by the practitioner attempting to assume what he/she "thinks" is going on, as opposed to what is actually the case.

Clearly, this system is a path toward resolution of a particular problem that has many branches or forks in the road, hence the importance of adhering to a logical plan of action. Make sure all attempts at treatment meet appropriate parameters of proper energetic logic and reason. In short, it all makes sense; it is the responsibility and requirement of the practitioner to have a sufficient understanding of the system to provide appropriate healing influence and avoid other less helpful activities.

Secondly, there are some pieces of equipment that are very useful. It must be stated at this point, that no equipment is absolutely necessary, as this can all be managed with the use of a proper and adequate philosophy and technical knowledge base and appropriately skilled use of the control of mind and sense of touch while performing the techniques involved. In the professional clinical setting, the "non-equipment" approach may be too time-consuming; so to address that issue, there is technology available that is well suited to this purpose. It should be noted that equipment is more useful for diagnostics than treatment, although both diagnosis and treatment are made more expedient with the use of proper equipment. Examples of equipment will be covered later on in this text.

USE OF THE HANDS AND THE MIND IN EMPLOYING THE CHALLENGE SYSTEM OF DISCOVERY

As briefly mentioned before, the hands of the practitioner are used to "challenge" specific meridians or acupuncture points for their suitability and involvement in specific conditions.

When the micro chakras of the fingertip pads are applied to the meridian or point, the only intention that the practitioner should have in mind is being curious as to whether this particular point or meridian is "reactive" or not...nothing else matters at this point. It's simply a yes or no inquiry.

To overcomplicate this technique can provide troublesome results, mostly by confusing the patient's system, the practitioner's sense of order, or both. Keep it simple. One of the likely complications I would expect to take place is the event of a student of the Eastern healing philosophies trying to figure out which finger to apply to a meridian or point based on its elemental polarity. This is neither necessary nor difficult to manage. Simply place the index finger pad or middle finger pad on the point of concern with the index and middle finger together, basically adjacent, with possibly both in contact with the point in question. It is not necessary to concern one's self with this.

The solution is as simple as not worrying about it and considering in your own mind (the practitioner's mind) that your fingers are functioning as a single, non-polar unit of investigation. Whether you believe it or not is of no real consequence. If that is your mindset, then that is what will happen. Keep it simple. The technique is to palpate the alarm point and the point of interest at the same time and get a "pain, less pain, no pain" reading and go with it. The complications come later when discerning the meridian interrelationships, if that is indeed necessary at all.

The simple reduction or absence of pain on the palpatory challenge is sufficient evidence that an energy-based condition does exist.

In the event that there appears to be a number of meridians involved, at that point, a careful consultation of the sheng and ko cycles and other relationships within the elemental system are definitely in order. To review this, please refer to the previous material titled How The Five Elements Interact to Create Balance and Imbalance beginning on page 155.

Attitude is an essential and fundamental component. Neutrality is in order, and no "pre-thinking" or guessing is to be exercised. As soon as the practitioner preconceives that he or she knows something and backs that up with any emotion at all (and personal conviction that something is the way one thinks it is, definitely qualifies as emotion), this will corrupt the evaluation and likely have poor results.

Question: How much pressure do I apply? Answer: Usually, not much. Moderation is important; so moderate and sometimes deep pressure is necessary at the alarm point, although only gentle touch for the purpose of communication with the point being challenged is necessary. Even holding the fingers near the skin where the point is located, and intending to be in communication with the point is often sufficient, especially if the practitioner also engages in advanced spiritual activities. This makes the healer's system even more powerful, conductive, and communicative. The most advanced and safe of these practices of which I am aware are found in Arhatic Yoga.

What about the patient being clothed? This issue is between the patient and the practitioner. Clothing covering the skin does not seem to present an impediment, but it is difficult to argue that skin to skin contact is not more conductive. One thing that must be considered is that the touch of the challenge must be light and gentle enough as to not constitute an acupressure treatment, only an investigative query. Another consideration is patient modesty and comfort.

If a patient is deeply concerned that their person is being invaded or their modesty compromised, their energy system will likely recoil and not be cooperative. It is essential to have an appropriate rapport and working relationship between the patient and the practitioner. In some instances, disrobing is a practical necessity in terms of accuracy of treatment. If the patient is very modest and this situation provides them with significant concern, there are other means of addressing their issues, such as Auriculotherapy or Ryodoraku. Neither of these modalities is likely to be offensive to anyone, as there is no contact or exposure of traditionally sensitive areas of the body.

HOW TO TELL IF A MERIDIAN IS TOO FULL OR TOO EMPTY

A meridian, chakra, nadi, or any other structure of the energy body may be too full or too empty, just the same as a container of water that is supposed to be "half full" when it is at its proper level of design and purpose.

First of all, in certain cases, the history will provide clues as to whether the meridian is too full or not. Generally, there is insufficient energy or corruption in the flow carried by a diseased meridian, but sometimes it is overfull.

The history of the problem is not only of primary importance in understanding what the practitioner is dealing with; but an abbreviated, but salient, history should be taken every time the patient is seen. Not only is this proper and standard professional health provider protocol, it is absolutely necessary. If you provided the corrective treatment during the last visit, the patient will have had some relief of their symptoms. If you only thought you provided corrective treatment, and the meridian or other energy structure were too full, then the patient would likely have their symptoms aggravated and worsened.

While this is an uncomfortable and sometimes unavoidable fact of practice, it is not such a terrible thing to have had happened. It is diagnostic. This is an impersonal function for the purpose of determining what needs to be done for the patient...it's about them. If the practitioner is distracted with personal issues or anything other than a sincere curiosity in terms of what the patient's problems is, it is time for the practitioner to withdraw for a moment or two and reacquire the necessary investigatory frame of mine. This said, practitioners are human beings with human concerns, so if there is some difficulty in determining the cause of the patient's problem, aside from possibly needing more data, some self-examination may reveal where the difficulty may be found. It's about the patient, so awareness (similar to "listening" and allowing information in) may be of more benefit than concentrating (similar to sending energy out) which is what a magnifying glass does with sunlight. Awareness (similar to listening) is how intuition works.

Rather than assume this is a black and white, right or wrong situation, there are times when it is very difficult to determine the full or empty status of a meridian. Besides that, contrary to the opinion of some schools of thought, a meridian may be both too full and too empty simultaneously in different places along the course of the meridian. It is no different than a river flowing along its course of a thousand miles. There may be drought at one end and a huge storm at the other or somewhere in between.

Another important factor not to be left out of the evaluation process is that of injury to a meridian. There are at least two types of ways in which a meridian may be injured (aside from emotional, chemical, or outside energetic pollution (as in with a homeopathic influence) which include what I term 'intention injury (extreme emotional effort resulting in an overload of the meridian without an accompanying physical injury)) and direct impact injury.

To aid in understanding of these principles, examples include: a young man came in to the clinic and was complaining of shoulder pain and weakness. The history of this was that he exerted a great deal of effort in order to move a very heavy object, which he was unable to move. He sustained what I term an intention injury of the large intestine meridian, and with the tonification of a single point along that meridian in the area of the shoulder, he was returned to normal immediately.

Another example was a woman of about sixty years who had attempted to lean against a wall, but the wall was farther from her than she realized, and she fell backward against it about 12 inches or so. She sustained an impact injury to her right bladder meridian, which caused right sided back pain for several years with the practice of hatha yoga being the only relief she could get, no matter how slight. Nothing else provided any benefit. Upon restoring the proper energy flow in her right bladder meridian, her pain was instantly relieved.

A third example, one injection of a vaccine into an acupuncture point of the large intestine meridian of the shoulder caused a pain that would not respond to normal care. Application of micro current to this point restored proper energy flow and the problem was relieved immediately. Intention, impact, and polluting injuries to meridians and their points appears to result in either partial or complete blockage of the energy flow, or at least a corruption to such flow. Actually, the most easily recognizable finding is that of increased pain on palpation of the alarm point, the challenged acupuncture point, or both. Referring back to the alarm point is one of the keys to understanding how this works.

Usually, both a meridian that is too full or too empty/corrupted is likely to elicit a painful response on palpation; but the too empty one will provide mild pain on palpation while the too full meridian will be very painful, possibly exquisitely painful at the slightest touch. In the event of this exquisite pain finding, immediately go to either the sedation point of the affected meridian or the opposing meridian's tonification point.

Don't mess around with lots of "diagnostic exercises" out of curiosity; just go to this simple procedure and get the patient out of pain. It is pretty much self-diagnostic, so all the other considerations are for "thought food." After the visit is over, the practitioner might attempt to discover the interrelationships involved. Complicated healing techniques often result in complications, so it is helpful to realize that most disease is actually simple in its origin and, therefore, simple in its resolution. There is great power in simplicity.

If you have someone screaming in pain on your treatment table, the meridian itself will indicate quite clearly which meridian is in trouble, especially with some gentle palpation. Then simply go to the sedation point and treat that as gently as possible. Don't mess around with all the technical paraphernalia you might have on hand; just sedate the meridian. On their next visit, do the technical stuff as it pleases you. This is a very simple situation, so don't complicate it while your patient suffers.

Now for the old and new in meridian evaluation: The old is what is known as pulse diagnosis, or pulse reading. One of my teachers in acupuncture once told me that there are probably only half a dozen acupuncturists in the world who can actually read pulses accurately. There are lots of schools of acupuncture and traditional Chinese medicine that attempt to teach this very fine art. In this age of science and proof of everything one does and says, pulse diagnosis is subjective to the person reading the pulse period.

It is subjective. The word "subjective" means it's changeable, open to interpretation, and not likely reproducible. Objective generally means it is not open to interpretation; and it means what it means, is not changeable, and is very reproducible.

On the other hand, there are other means of discovery that are both objective and commonly available. Ryodoraku is one of these. It is an electronic means of evaluating the character of the acupuncture meridians and uses some of the same points as pulse reading uses. It is reproducible and objective. Of course, like any other technique, it must be done properly.

There is an electronic unit that is available to the public called the Electro Meridian Imaging (EMI) system. It comes in several models designed for the different levels of practitioners and technical levels that some practitioners prefer. Its main use, in my opinion, is that of sorting out difficult and complicated cases. Examples of these types of cases include fibromyalgia, some migraine headaches, instances where a patient has several conditions overlapping one another, those "mystery" cases, and patients who are not conscious, or are in a coma.

When this technology is taken to one of its further extremes, it involves the use of computerized and computer-embodied systems that do extremely detailed and delicate energetic comparisons and evaluations. Usually these rely on acupuncture points found near the proximal corners of the fingernails, called tsing points. This is usually quite a bit removed from the practices this book mainly concerns itself with; so it is the very expensive and technical equipment we are not including in our considerations. The term commonly applied to these expensive systems is "electro-dermal screening" and is employed by advanced nutritional practitioners.

TONIFYING AND SEDATING - TIME AND PLACE

Generally, when a meridian is found to be too empty or there is corruption within its energies, it requires rectification. To help understand this, some elementary fluid dynamics are in order. A fluid that is turbulent does not flow evenly or at its appropriate rate. In other words, it goes in more directions than appropriate; therefore, not enough arrives at its proper destination. This translates directly to "too empty", as not enough energy is getting there to do the intended job.

Considering that the central theme in the meridian and chakra systems is balance, and when the imbalance occurs, the goal is the proper restoration of that state of balance. This has direct aspects, indirect aspects, and exceptions.

Since emptiness is usually the case, when in doubt, tonify. Always make an effort to recognize whether the condition is one of emptiness or of being too full; but if that is not possible, as may be the case if electronic diagnostic means are not available, assume the channel is empty and tonify.

Of course, if it is found that the meridian is discovered to be too full, sedation is in order.

The question of how long to apply the treatment depends on the type of practice employed. In traditional acupuncture with needles being the mode of treatment, a certain number of minutes is used for tonification (with the intention of tonification in the mindset of the practitioner) and twice that amount of time for sedation (with the intention of sedation in the mindset of the practitioner) with the addition of "wiping closed" the point after the needle is withdrawn with a stroking motion of the practitioner's finger against the point.

In Auriculotherapy, which is typically a micro-current mediated practice, 8 seconds is for tonification and 16 or 32 seconds is used for sedation. Again, the intention the practitioner holds in mind is important. This conformity and congruence of mind and action helps provide for a more coherent and effective treatment.

The previously referred to exceptions to the time a point is treated is especially applicable to Auriculotherapy. Certain conditions and certain points warrant more time than would be otherwise deemed appropriate. The lung points may be energized for as long a time as several minutes in cases of smoking cessation or asthma and the anti-depression point may be energized for nearly as long. In the phase II system, sometimes these points may be energized for several minutes with intermittent queries to the patient about the status of their pain. This is usually a technique employed in cases of chronic pain and is an advanced level of practice.

When applying pranic healing to a condition, the terms tonification and sedation are not used; instead, this system uses the terms energize rather than tonify, and sweep or cleanse rather than sedate. Usually, in the case of pranic healing, the practitioner is already trained in that art; plus the books written by Grand Master Choa Kok Sui, the founder and developer of Modern Pranic Healing are very detailed and complete, so simply looking up the technique in the book and simply following the protocols given will provide the proper guidance.

I very strongly recommend that people interested in using purely energy healing methods be properly trained and take the appropriate classes in Pranic Healing before attempting to use that practice. Pranic Healing is a foundational healing art that tends to support all other systems when done properly.

Before embarking on any modality of healing, make sure all possible and appropriate training has been acquired. Consider someone who takes their automobile to someone at a tire shop for an engine rebuild. Typically, this worker is not adequately qualified.

Sometimes the questions of voltage, amperage, and frequency arise when the topic of micro-current is discussed. The basic frequency for the human body is 10 hertz (10 pulses per second). In Auriculotherapy, there are many frequencies; but the basic one is still 10 cycles per second. Voltage and amperage come in a distant second place in importance after frequency.

The main concern with amperage is for the pure and simple reason that too much amperage causes pain. This is not a "no pain, no gain" system of treatment. In fact, it is designed to be so painless and gentle, that the patient is hardly aware of having had anything done to them. This is one of my definitions that applies to "the perfect treatment"…painlessness, effectiveness, and non-invasiveness. It is like the concept of a very small key opening the lock of a very large door. Power is not necessary.

HOW MUCH IS ENOUGH?

HOW MUCH IS TOO MUCH?

WHEN TO QUIT

These are questions that are complicated to answer, but appear as simple questions.

Enough is the amount required to neutralize the challenge finding. What this means is that when the patient's system has all it needs for balancing, the alarm point will cease to be tender on palpation. Sometimes it never quite resolves due to complicating factors, but the most appropriate choice should be one of conservative treatment and simplicity. It is possible to chase problems throughout a person's entire system, but that is wholly problematic for lots of reasons...don't do it. You may create more imbalances than you're attempting to correct. The system has self-correcting mechanisms built into it, so give the system a chance to do what it is designed to do. Time is required for the assimilation of the treatment. This is a conservative type of treatment, so be conservative.

How much is too much? When you have treated more than a reasonable number of points on a meridian, say, more than 10 or 12, and the same number of points applies to Auriculotherapy, you may confuse the patient's system. If you are treating a bilateral condition, such as dysmenorrhea or irritable bowel syndrome, where both the right and left stomach meridians are involved, then you can double that number, although the number of points per side is usually only 7. During each subsequent visit/treatment, re-challenging each point is usually not required.

After a reasonable period of gaining experience, the practitioner will have developed a sense of what to treat for a certain condition. Do not use shortcuts, like treating only the master points on the ear and then sending the patient home. That does not address the condition at the depth necessary to achieve a proper resolution. Do it right. By that I mean to do the master points after doing the anatomical and functional points associated with the specific condition, which is also evidenced by the readings the micro-current device provides (presuming you are using a device of adequate sophistication, which can be expensive).

In terms of timing between treatments, there is a lot yet to be discovered. It is often a good idea to have the patient return on a weekly basis. Is this a guess? Sure it is. It takes time for the patient's system to assimilate the changes you have induced. Of course, they are advised to pay attention to what is taking place within them and to come back sooner if necessary, but come back in a week regardless. A major reason for this is what is termed the "subclinical condition". What this is, is the level an imbalance may exist on that is beneath the level of the awareness of the patient or before testing can reveal it. Sometimes the patient will simply feel a little better and figure that is all the better they will get considering they may have had the problem for years. If they have had the problem for years, usually a longer treatment schedule will be in order, but not always.

The subclinical condition is basically lying in wait until it gets the opportunity to express itself as a full blown condition. This can be prevented by proper case management. Remember, that while you may seem to be the local fire department, putting out people's "fires", is most certainly an inadequate treatment system just waiting to ruin your reputation as a quality practitioner.

As a preventive effort in my own practice, I have told patients who were not adhering to their treatment plan, that if they did not make a substantially better effort, they should seek another doctor. Not following good advice will result in them not getting well, and people might assume it is the practitioner not doing their job correctly, and so their reputation would be harmed through no fault of their own. Of course, this was a threat I offered to only the worst offenders.

When a combination of the patient having no symptoms, the alarm points not being tender, and all systems functioning at their proper level, it is then that care should be spaced out to two, three, or four times the normal interval between visits. The reason for follow up visits is to ensure that their system is actually in balance. This is not always an easy thing to ascertain due to the dynamic nature of the individual and the possibility that they are not still exposed to the causative factors that created the problem in the first place.

Balance is the key. Being aggressive is problematic. In this practice, a large ego is not your friend. Be thoughtful and gentle. Be conservative and curious. It's not about you the practitioner, but the restoration of balance to the patient's compromised system…period.

WHEN NOT TO START – ARE YOU IN OVER YOUR HEAD?

To be sure, this is a difficult situation from beginning to end.

There are those cases that defy one's abilities. In the health care professions we see those special individuals to whose condition is applied the term "train wreck". If you imagine each part of the human system as an individual car of a long railway train and this train is in a massive wreck, which derails all, or many, of the cars, this is how the person's system is. It is like these railway cars – most of them are still containing their cargo, but they are not able to perform the rest of their normal function. It is a loosely applied but fairly accurate analogy.

Additionally, these people know they are "train wreck" people, accept that as fact, and usually they expect the practitioner to do all the work for a problem that does not belong to the practitioner. Beyond that, there is so much wrong with them that if something were actually fixed, the intensity of the rest of their problems would make the positive changes nearly unnoticeable. Usually these are what might be called "derelict cases" that the conventional system did not know how to manage, therefore, mismanaged them to an extreme extent then left them on their own, often after draining the patients of most of their financial resources in the process.

And then...on top of all that, these patients very often do not comply with the very life-saving instruction you sent them home with. It's "doctor, please help me.", and not "how can I help myself?" I'm not even going to go into the dietary abyss into which they usually have thrown themselves.

That does not mean you cannot help them; only that most often, it is a very long and unrewarding journey back to health for them...and for you. These are the cases that test your grip on sanity.

The mechanics of this situation are that the damage is done, and done so broadly and deeply that it requires the most resolute and self-disciplined of souls to dig their way out of the abyss. Usually, their dietary requirements are extremely narrow and strict. It is a situation that must be attacked on nearly every front imaginable.

This type of patient is becoming more common and is difficult to treat. Generally, the ideal patient is the one who is just sick and tired of being sick and tired or the one who has just found out they have such and such disease, say, diabetes and want to be rid of it as soon as possible because they understand the fate that awaits them.

It is these cases that are the most rewarding to work with. The train wreck ones, while the prospect of winning their battle is a tempting challenge, may be more than a match for the healer; as the therapist tends to adopt people's problems if they are around them long enough – then, it's the practitioner's problem too. Then the practitioner is in over his or her head for sure.

The next type of patient is the one that has been in misery for years; all the conventional ideas have been tried, and all the "normal" tests have been run and found to be within normal parameters. Usually, this is a case heaven sent to the energy practitioner, as the conventional system has done a pretty thorough screening for physically-based problems, and that can usually be trusted in doing that very well. Sometimes the person has really in-depth issues that seem to have no means of resolution regardless of how many times you have evaluated them via Ryodoraku or other means.

Often, they have some very deep internal issue that may be genetic, some sort of miasm (inherited genetic-like condition), some past life, or karmic issue of immense intensity. These are possible to extract, but access to the timeless component within the patient's energy structure is required. Obviously, this is very advanced work.

There are those difficulties that, after you practice long enough, you will encounter that cannot be fixed....not by your hand anyway. After realizing you are baffled, stop wasting both your time and the patients' time and have a meaningful consultation about why the two of you should either continue or cease treatment. Sometimes your care actually gives them enough help, although not complete or enough to brag about; it is enough to continue receiving treatment and experiencing adequate appreciable benefit.

This is not to be confused with the entrenched, chronic disease pattern such as an old case of Crohn's disease, where the tissues have become so degraded and atrophied that long-term and continual care is necessary. This is not a train wreck case so do your best to not confuse an entrenched case with a nearly impossible one, though they may seem very much alike – and possibly are; but the entrenched one is solvable.

HOW LONG WILL A BALANCING OR TREATMENT LAST?

That depends on a number of factors. These include: the knowledge and skill of the practitioner, the condition of the patient, the length of time the condition has existed, the lifestyle of the patient, the compliance with the practitioner's professional advice - assuming that such advice is good and proper advice, the complexity of the problem, and external factors the patient may be subject to (for example, family members, friends, and others who may offer differing advice, whether it's good advice or not. If it interferes, it interferes.)

If the skill exercised by the practitioner is less than optimal, the condition will return to its previous level more quickly than if a more complete treatment had been rendered. If the treatment were overdone, keeping in mind that this whole affair is one of balance, it would be expected that untoward changes may develop or a new condition be created. While this is possible, it is generally unlikely due to the inherent self-correcting nature of the energetic system itself. If too long an interval between treatments elapses, the condition "re-imbalances" itself and the symptoms return to their old status.

Treatment frequency can be compared to attempting to sweep water up an incline with a broom. If swept often enough, the water will be propelled over the crest of the incline; but if too long a period elapses between sweeps, the water returns to, or toward, its original starting point.

When a patient reports that, although you scheduled them to return in one week, the symptoms returned in two days, at that point, they should be advised that their condition is more acute than originally suspected and reschedule them for three times a week for at least one, probably two weeks. After that, try twice a week.

One consideration must be made in such circumstances, which is to question them in regard to adherence to the lifestyle advice that was given them. The situation will usually work out to be that either they have not made the fundamental lifestyle adjustments they were advised to make, which is a sign of inadequate patient education, lack of compliance, or their condition is actually more deeply rooted and severe than originally suspected.

It can be said that if someone does not alter the unhealthy lifestyle that created the condition in the first place, how can the continuance of that lifestyle be expected to have a productive outcome? The changes in style of living that are advised by the wise practitioner are not to be either given or taken lightly.

If the patient's home or work environment has within it destructive factors, this can derail even the best of treatments for a number of reasons. If the patient's spouse is troublesome, a smoker, insists on an unhealthy diet and ridicules the patient about the necessary changes, or there are many other factors, this can present problematic influences beyond the control of the practitioner.

If there is an honest lack of funds such that treatment cannot be managed, I would advise treating this patient anyway. Having them promise to send in other potential patients who are able and willing to pay your fee is a relatively safe bet to make, although it is usually the patient who cannot pay that associates with others in a similar financial condition. This may be more of a moralistic statement than a practical one.

WHAT CAUSES A PROBLEM TO COME BACK OR BECOME WORSE?

In short, either the patient has experienced some sort of trauma (physical, mental, emotional, social, environmental, or spiritual), the practitioner did something wrong, or something very pathologic buried deep within the patients' system was uncovered by the work previously done.

In the event of additional factors, another history is in order, making sure to include all of the items included above: physical, mental, emotional, social, environmental, and spiritual. Often, they cannot initially identify what it was that traumatized them. They may be advised to think about it and call back when it occurs to them what had happened that they could not think of while at the office. Most of the time, they will realize what it was.

The practitioner should be able to guide them in their self-examination by the emotional patterns characteristic for each element of the system. The way to manage this is by recognizing the affected meridian and advising them to look for something that happened that would match up with that character of pathologic emotion.

Next is the issue of the practitioner making some sort of mistake in his or her evaluation or treatment. While this is a bad thing to have happen, it does occur from time to time and usually when the practitioner does not properly "follow" the case. When the practitioner pushes ahead with their ego or "standard treatment" in a unique case, they are usually going in the wrong direction and may complicate things even further.

What does one do about it? First of all, the knowledge that an unnecessary problem exists is in order...without going into great detail about it. Something might have been missed. That's simple and common enough. What to do about it is start all over from the beginning...the very beginning. Review the history in great detail, as something vitally important was probably missed, either due to the practitioner being in too big a hurry, the questions asked being inadequate either in number or detail, or the patient not having a clear memory. Don't bother assigning blame; it's not worth the effort and only causes problems; just get to work and do it both carefully and thoroughly. Between the two of you, it can usually be sorted out the second time around; but no one likes the first time around when it's wrong...ever.

The aura of a person functions somewhat like their skin...it keeps the inside in, the outside out, and prevents the two from mixing inappropriately. If your skin has enough tears in it that it cannot keep the inside in and the outside out, you have a major problem and your health will be greatly altered. The aura, when torn by some event, sometimes as the result of psychic attack, no matter how much healing energy is put in by the healer, it will simply pour right back out, leaving the victim weak, feeling very lifeless, and usually in a state of deep and pervasive depression.

In cases such as these, a skilled and powerful energy healer sufficient to the task of mending the aura is required. Before that healer can do their work properly, it must be known that a torn aura is indeed present. No substantial healing can be realized in cases such as this without the aura having been repaired, as that person's life energy simply pours out of their system nearly as fast as it is put in and disperses into the environment. The victims of this condition are perpetually "empty" and feel that way, although no "scientific or medical tests" will reveal the problem.

Sometimes there is hidden a very pathologic thing that you may unwittingly release from its organic prison. When you have energetically pried the lid off something truly scary, it's time to read the segment on page 182 of when not to start. If you are not highly skilled in clairvoyance and exorcism, you may well be in over your head. It's helpful to have people in your circle of friends who have these rare talents that can help you out.

The corollary to "when not to start" once you have already started is to quit. Running like the devil is after you is not helpful. Regardless of the movies you have seen and the stories you have heard, or even not heard, spiritual possession is real. There is a good and not-so-bad part to this. Well, the good part is actually bad; it's just not as bad as the bad part, so here's the "good" part. Usually "things" like this end up in a person's system for a reason, and you are not the reason.

These things have consciousness and like to consume energy and have usually established some sort of parasitic relationship with the host/patient. Once discovered, it or they (usually "they") will usually throw a small tantrum and go back to its normal lifestyle if left alone. If you mess with this it/them excessively, they may cause more trouble than you might be prepared or able to deal with. Just leave it alone if you are not a number of things, namely: spiritually protected, highly spiritually developed, skilled at exorcism, have both experience and confidence, and are truly clairvoyant. If any of these necessary qualifications are weak or absent and you mess with some malevolent possessing intruder, you yourself may be its next meal/victim.

Don't let your ego get either your patient or yourself in hot water. Remember that the patient may have been living with this thing in them for decades and got along relatively well, all things considered, before you showed up and disturbed it. It is a truly rare event to run into something that would require the response of "run like hell", so don't overreact.

If, for some reason, you find this book too spooky for you, put down the book and go back to your former pretend lifestyle and stay away from the inside of other people's energy being; you are not qualified to enter therein, mainly by default.

PART SEVEN

HOW TO MANAGE THE VERY COMPLICATED CASE

This is where the real work begins. In these cases the history must be as in-depth, detailed, and thorough as possible. Every detail must be considered on as many of the following levels as possible: physical, chemical, old injury, toxic scar, emotional, mental, karmic, and spiritual, including having possibly been spiritually attacked or possessed. If, in your personal style of faith, you believe that these things do not happen, remember, this is not about you; and please don't allow what you don't believe to limit your service to others. What if you are wrong? If you are wrong, then the patient may suffer due to your ignorance.

In the history, consider that the person may have had Lyme disease, nicknamed "the great imitator" due to its ability to mimic a great number of diseases. It is always a good idea to screen for this disease, as it seems more common than most health professionals suspect; and since the conventional medical system has proven very ineffective in dealing with it, they generally try to avoid bringing up the subject unless the situation forces the issue.

The best diagnostic test available for Lyme disease is not completely reliable, so it is a good idea to use your own means to evaluate for this very insidious and destructive micro-organism. Whether one uses muscle-testing (Applied Kinesiology style), pendulum, or any other reliable means of discovery one may have at their disposal, do it. If you are wrong, and believe that the patient has Lyme disease, and they do not, the treatments commonly used in alternative healing would likely be useful anyway, plus such treatments are quite safe.

There are several treatments that come to mind that appear to be effective in the resolution of Lyme disease. These are MMS (activated 28% sodium chlorite solution), Rife frequency generator, and the Life Vessel. I'm sure there are others, so consider this the short list. A homeopathic nosode may be useful, but I have not heard of that as a consideration for Lyme disease. On another note, sometimes tissue toxicity may be mistaken for Lyme disease; but again, the usual treatments have a detoxifying effect as part of their natural function. What if the patient has Lyme disease and you do not find out? This is a recipe for unending health problems for that patient.

With all the above considerations having been managed, one major consideration must be dealt with. In these "train wreck" cases, the elemental, sheng and ko cycle dynamic equilibrium is usually thrown far out of balance. I liken this to a ball of yarn that the cat has played with for some time – the patient's energy system being represented by the tangled ball of yarn. You are almost certain to be both wrong and misled by attempting to name a "named diagnostic entity", which is nearly impossible.

The point to this is that one must untangle one knot at a time. The method I use is Ryodoraku. I use the Electro Meridian

Imaging (EMI) protocol, which simply helps me balance the elemental, sheng, and ko cycle components on a real-time, current-status, basis. I call it "the great unraveller", because it has the capacity to show the character of disorder that must be re-ordered.

In any complicated or complex case, it is wise to employ methodology that serves to bring to light the hidden aspects of a patient's problems. Other methods include pulse diagnosis, reading the auricle of the ear, Applied Kinesiology, and others. The reason I utilize Ryodoraku as a primary tool of investigation is because it presents a comprehensive picture of the entire meridian system, which is foundational to nearly all definitive health problems.

Patience, mostly on the part of the patient is paramount. Additionally, the practitioner should not try to do too much at one time. These patients are fragile, out of balance in ways difficult to imagine, toxic, and often do not have the lifestyle habits conducive to healing.

A gentle, comprehensive approach is in order. Dietary changes are usually not well tolerated; so a gradual shift in diet, the addition of digestive enzymes, probiotics, and gentle exercise are often a good start that can be managed by these types of patients. It is helpful to remember that, in most cases, it isn't that they cannot make big changes, but they will not make big changes. Consider that if they had a really good lifestyle already in place, they would not be in this shape to begin with. If they claim that they do, upon further investigation, it is usually found that they don't but only think they do.

The use of a huge regimen of dietary supplements, while often the style of many practitioners, will usually overwhelm the patient both ideologically and financially; and they may fall away from care. It is good practice to work with the patient, not on the patient. Likewise, the patient should be working with the practitioner.

When practicing in the world of alternative care, often it is these complex cases that are seen. This is due to the tendency of people to seek conventional care first; and after that does not work, usually for far too long a period, they seek the alternative care out of desperation....which is usually where they should have been in the first place.

PRANIC HEALING, PRANIC PSYCHOTHERAPY, CRYSTALS AND THEIR USES: PURE ENERGY

There are two basic forms of existence that make up our world, physical matter and energy. Both exist in many states of being. Physical matter is found in solid, liquid, and gaseous states; and the terms we use for spiritual energy include emotional, mental, and spiritual or causal. In "normal life" in our society, the two seem to be disconnected and separate, but they are not. There is a fourth state of physical matter that is not often discussed called plasma. This seems more spiritual than physical to most people due to it not being apparent to our senses. It bridges the gap, so to speak, between the physical and spiritual levels of our world.

The concept of prana in terms of definitions and discussion is treading a slippery slope indeed, as there are many interpretations of what prana actually is, plus the fact that there are many kinds of prana. To begin a discourse on this topic, it would seem appropriate to start at the top and work downward, so to speak. This is actually unnecessary due to the fact that the simple understanding that there are many kinds of prana that exist regardless of what we believe or call it.

The Christian term for prana is Holy Spirit; and this often has been defined, or actually not been defined very well, on a historical basis. It is easier for our purposes to stick to the use of the word "prana", so the confusion that may otherwise take place does not. (The Holy Spirit, in some cases, refers primarily to divine energy with consciousness. However, this energy flows through all of us and becomes regular prana as it is processed through the human system.)

Prana has its beginning near the apex of the Creative process and differentiates and "devolves" into more diffuse and dense forms as the process progresses, ending in the creation of physical matter. It is for this reason prana is such an effective means of enabling physical healing.

The meridian, chakra, and nadi systems all deal with prana in much the same way as our physical bodies deal with air, food, and water. It should be remembered what prana is to physical matter is like what steam is to water. While inherently of similar nature, the prana is not nearly as dense as physical matter; so like steam is with water, it takes a LOT of steam to produce a little water; so also does it take a LOT of prana to produce a little physical matter or physical result. This will then bring one to the facts of the matter of just how well can one connect with the Source of prana and how able are they to conduct that prana in their healing practice.

Connection and conduction are the two primary concepts in practicing energy medicine. A short cut we use is micro-current that is very, very similar to pranic energies but is much more "condensed" and is readily available for clinical use. Prana can be very subtle; while in comparison, electricity is quite dense, thereby enabling the practitioner to provide effective treatment while not forcing him or her to have spent years and years in mystical studies and yogic practices simply to enable them to be effective clinically.

Pranic healing is the science and art of determining the presence of inharmonious life energies, extracting from the patients' systems these diseased energies, and replacing them with healthy harmonious energies. These energies, both of disease and healing, can take many forms; but to keep it simple is sufficient for our purposes. Training and literature on this topic are readily available from the pranic healing groups that can be found globally.

I consider pranic healing a central component in one's arsenal of healing knowledge and skills. It is probably the most comprehensive and complete system available for educating one in the area of energy disease and the use of energy in the restoration of health. It presents a complete and balanced knowledge base and set of concepts such that the subtle areas of concern addressed in this book may be more easily understood regarding the various energetic imbalances a patient may have.

Crystal Healing

Crystal healing, including pranic crystal healing, has been around for many thousands of years. Crystals or gemstones can be very effective when used in healing...and also very expensive. There are some ways to reduce the expenses involved once one is educated in the properties of certain crystals.

Crystals were commonly used in radios for defining and managing frequency. When diseased, one's energy frequencies are outside their proper parameters; and when in a good state of health, their frequencies are within those parameters. This can easily be understood with the concept of radio frequencies, that crystals can be employed in "frequency management." When the frequency is off, accurate communication does not take place.

Crystals may not have a brain; but they can be directed to perform as they otherwise, in their natural state, would not. Due to the very fact that they exist, therefore they have a state of being; they are actually beings. While inanimate, their "beingness" cannot be argued, plus the fact that they are capable of conforming to conditioning. This conditioning can take two basic forms, physical (size, shape, and purity) and energetic (connection, conduction, and intention) – and, yes, they can be programmed (remember things). If they did not have these qualities, they would never have been considered for tools of healing in the first place.

Quartz. Quartz is relatively cheap and is very programmable. In pranic crystal healing, the crystal is energetically purified, programmed, and consecrated. Its abilities are expanded such that it can perform or mimic to a great (and to a practical) extent the qualities found in its other crystalline relatives. The crystal functions to focus, amplify, and draw in greater amounts of the right kind of energies for the cleansing and healing process. It also serves to protect the healer from "backlash" from certain types of problems patients might have; as anything escaping the patient, or being extracted, is stopped by the crystal and not transferred to the healer's hands. Crystals serve to make the whole healing experience more effective and efficient.

Again, I would strongly advise that anyone seriously interested in the use of crystals in healing be trained in the pranic crystal healing methods developed by Grand Master Choa Kok Sui of the Philippines. These are modern practices; but when one searches the bookstores for crystal healing material, there is much folklore and legend incorporated in what is found.

The pranic healing system was developed in a very scientific and logical manner based on frequencies and what these frequencies actually do. The developer, Master Choa Kok Sui, was a chemical engineer and was very careful in the development of his methods and incorporated many years of research and testing to insure that his material was both accurate and practical. Having known him personally, I can attest to his thoroughness and accuracy.

While a number of methods can be utilized in crystal healing, the style of practice of the healer would be the determining factor in the crystals required. If one were to specifically be a crystal healer, and perform mainly "laying on of stones", this too can be managed with various types of quartz. Pranic crystal healing is a very flexible system of healing.

Crystals make the whole job of energy healing more powerful, efficient, and safe; but care must be exercised so not to exceed the patients' tolerance of things they may not understand, or possibly regard as something to be feared or avoided, usually due to religious concerns. To be sure, this has nothing to do with witchcraft. Crystals simply manage energy and frequencies.

In pranic psychotherapy, usually a crystal is used mainly for its ability to go deeply into the chakras of the patient and protect the healer from the thought-forms and disease-causing emotional influences being extracted. In any event, pranic psychotherapy is the removal of negative psychological influences that are either "foreign" (are from outside the patients' system but are now "infecting" their chakras or other parts of their energy body) or "domestic" (have been generated from within and are still present and are negatively influencing the patient).

These "psychological entities" seem to have a life of their own and alter the inner tranquility of the individual on both conscious and subconscious levels often resulting in the sabotage of the individual's best intentions. The people with these problems seem to be in otherwise good condition but sabotage themselves for some reason. These infective entities are the cause of the "wrecked life" in the absence of physically observed disease.

Often, these subtle forms of influence are from either a past incarnation or have been generated by an abusive relationship in the current incarnation, usually a parent, sibling, teacher, bully, life circumstances, or even the media. There are forms of psychic attack that are capable of causing these things to take place. Regardless of what caused the influence of interest to be present, it can be removed. Care must be exercised, especially in long term cases, that the patient out of habit does not recreate the problem. Usually, creating an entirely new and better, more positive, lifestyle is the best solution.

Here is a very short story to serve as an example: I once listened as a concerned student asked the Teacher how to change the future. The Teacher was taken aback by the complexity of the concern. He simply replied, "It is much easier to create a new future than change the original one." This is the style of advice I propose, changing the whole lifestyle to a much better one; as when one attempts to patch up a wrecked lifestyle, what they often end up with is a patched wrecked lifestyle. It is still wrecked; so change the whole thing – the diet, thinking patterns, activities – the whole thing – ponder that.

In the last analysis, everything physical is made of energy, only in a slower vibrating form, at lower frequency. The relationship is one of density; the more dense the more physical and the less dense the more spiritual. It is a very definite scale of densities and frequencies in a complete spectrum. When these frequencies and energies are disrupted or corrupted in some fashion, disease is created. This is the Law of Creation in action.

Every disease is created by the Law of Nature for very specific reasons. Nothing happens without a cause, and the cause determines the effect. In the case of disease, we often wail and cry "How did I get this?" or "Why me?" but there is always a reason. Forget the drama that society is so distracted with. It's a waste of both time and energy, therefore, impractical. Did you deserve whatever that problem was? Who knows? The point is that a specific problem could not have happened without its specific cause.

There are innumerable forms and styles of energy healing. The reason I choose pranic healing as my prime example is that, after 30 years of trying other things plus the fact that I was incorporating this into a clinical practice, it is the only one that I found fits me on a practical and effective level.

If you are a busy practitioner in the laying on of crystals or gemstones and you have four or more patient stations in your establishment, then treatment time is not such a concern; but such is not likely the case. In this book I am going to presume that you see patients one at a time; therefore, some level of expediency and practicality is required. When all is taken into consideration that is presented herein as proper practice, scheduling is enough of a challenge without complicating it further. Practice style is very individual.

RYODORAKU: THE GREAT UNRAVELLER

Ryodoraku has its roots in the Japanese healing arts. Ryodoraku was developed in 1950 by Yoshio Nakatani, M.D., Ph.D., as he was measuring the electrical resistance of acupuncture points in a patient. Without going in to great detail, Dr. Nakatani found that the Source (yuan) points were the most conductive and were the most effective for measuring Qi (chi, prana, life force) within the meridian in question. Also, it was very useful for both diagnosis and treatment.

From this was developed the system that incorporates electro-meridian imaging (EMI), which I use much of the time for evaluating the energy-based problems of my patients, particularly the more serious or complex ones. In a simple case of migraine or irritable bowel syndrome, often I do not use EMI; but in cases of fibromyalgia and other complex cases, it is indispensible.

Ryodoraku is the practice of measuring the electrical conductivity of the Source (yuan) acupuncture points on the hands, wrists, feet, and ankles. These particular points are very stable in their behavior in the indication of the status of the entire acupuncture meridian system. The readings are then graphed, either manually or electronically, to produce a meaningful representation of the condition of each of the 24 classical meridians. When the acupuncture system is in a chaotic, or very complicated pathological state, Ryodoraku is invaluable in determining what is to be done at the present time. In classic traditional acupuncture, pulse diagnosis was used to make these determinations.

According to my acupuncture teacher, himself a Master Acupuncturist, there are likely less than a dozen practitioners world-wide who can match the accuracy of the Ryodoraku system. In pulse diagnosis, there are 28 different, named, distinct pulses the practitioner must be able to 'read' accurately, and this skill level is very rare indeed, hence Ryodoraku to the rescue. With Ryodoraku, any reasonably competent practitioner can obtain the information required for treatment as would the few masters of pulse diagnosis.

The EMI system has a number of more and less complex iterations, depending on how automated, computerized, or simple it is. Some units have only the ability of evaluation, while others incorporate treatment capabilities. It should be noted that if evaluating an acupuncture point for any longer than 2 or 3 seconds, it may corrupt the accuracy of the evaluation; so be brief lest you "muddy the very water you are attempting to see through" by unintentionally performing a treatment. The evaluation process introduces energy into the point, so it has the potential of performing treatment when your intention is evaluation.

By recording or writing down and comparing the electrical values obtained with EMI, it becomes very evident where the difficulties lie with any given patient. This is especially so when using the EMI computer generated bar graph that is available, and usually is included with the purchase of a new unit. For licensed practitioners of medicine, chiropractic, etc., there are no limitations regarding these purchases; but for the not traditionally licensed alternative provider, only the "non-treatment" models may be available.

For my own use, while I have the model that is capable of treatment, I don't use it for treatment due to the fact that I have a different unit that is both easier and of more gentle character than the EMI unit...and also much more expensive. It should be noted that the amount of electrical current and voltage is not that great; so a very mild current, regardless of voltage (particularly if its pulse rate is 10 cycles per second), will work just fine. It should also be noted that anytime the energy body is brought into balance, the patient will benefit; and this is probably the most reliable means for establishing this primary balance. It is easy to learn and practice, plus, it is not invasive to the patients' privacy; as only the hands, wrists, feet, and ankles are exposed or contacted.

AURICULOTHERAPY: THE MICROCOMPUTER KEYBOARD OF THE SYSTEM, A FINE ART

Auriculotherapy is the treatment of disease by utilizing the auricle of the ear as an access medium to the patients' systems on both physical and energetic levels.

To the reader who has knowledge of classic Chinese ear acupuncture, there are some things that are noteworthy. The old Chinese system was a grouping of both anatomical and functional points that was skewed toward the direction of the energetic part of the patient.

In the 1950's, a French neurologist named Claude Nogier noticed some interesting scars on some of this patients' ears that were an alternative treatment for sciatica. As Dr. Nogier further investigated the ear, he noticed that there were distinct electrical properties to the ear; and these characteristics were distributed in a pattern of reflex points that were along embryonic tissue patterns, dividing the ear into specific "anatomical" regions.

As Dr. Nogier's investigations continued, he discovered an "inverted fetus" type of pattern to these points and organ locations. He then presented this to the Chinese acupuncture community in China, who were very open to his findings. In fact, they were so interested in this material that they initiated a several-yearlong study of Auriculotherapy, thus furthering the development of this art of healing.

Due to these developments, there are two distinct, but overlapping, styles of Auriculotherapy. Many of the points are shared between the two systems and many are not. The European method originated by Dr. Nogier leans toward the more physical aspects of Auriculotherapy. The Chinese method leans toward the more energetic aspects of Auriculotherapy.

In classic Chinese-style body acupuncture, the points provide a very polar influence on the patient. This may have wonderful results; or if the practitioner treats the patient utilizing the wrong points, a bad situation may be made worse. This is the fear of every practitioner. In Auriculotherapy, the points have a "normalizing" effect. There is less concern about mixing up the strategies of tonifying and sedating. Usually, making a mistake has no effect – unless the practitioner goes far out of his or her way to cause problems.

With that being said, Auriculotherapy is "nearly bulletproof" in terms of patient safety. In fact, even when done wrong, it usually provides benefit plus the fact that this is one modality of treatment that can be "put into place on Monday". This means that after the first seminar, the practitioner can be effective as soon as he or she returns to the office. All they have to do is just look up the problem in the book and treat the points indicated therein...if they have a positive reading with the instrument.

If one considers the utility and central purpose of the keyboard to the modern computer (without the consideration of voice recognition software), this single component of the system represents the most accessible and capable means of managing the entire system.

The energy body is extremely complex, with the auricle (outer flap) of the ear serving as an access point and control mechanism, much as a keyboard for a computer. Through this mechanism, we have a very, very effective means of aid in the balancing of the system on the inside such that the outer, physical, is balanced.

The auricle of the ear is a micro-system that renders us capable of both simple diagnosis and treatment, much like foot reflexology. In my opinion, Auriculotherapy is by far the most comprehensive and accessible of systems. Each ear contains over 200 individual reflex points. Proper equipment is encouraged as is the use of micro-current and a unit sufficiently developed that it will reveal to the practitioner in a very precise way the electrical status of the reflex point under consideration.

Acupuncture needles may be used; but in my professional opinion, this style of treatment falls short in terms of actual, practical point evaluation. Treatment can be much better managed when using a quality micro-current system. I have been practicing and instructing in Auriculotherapy for nearly 20 years and have formed my opinions accordingly.

To address some of the capacity possessed by the ear, the physical auricle of the ear is innervated by the three major components of the physical nervous system: the cranial nerves, the autonomic nerves, and the spinal nerves. These are related physically and physiologically to every tissue in the body. There are also relationships with the energetic components. In the European style of Auriculotherapy, there is a complete system of interrelating points that encompasses the duration of a problem, organ, tissue, and cellular levels of concern and accessibility. No other Auriculotherapy system does this. To the conscientious practitioner, this represents a central modality of evaluation and treatment.

Auriculotherapy is one of the best pain management tools available. When patients come in with those "mystery pains" that no other practitioner has been able to resolve, Auriculotherapy may well provide the solution. It's great for working with chemical addictions too. I use it exclusively for asthma and other conditions of a "functional" nature. In patients whose personality does not permit access to certain body areas, Auriculotherapy can usually manage the situation very well.

Auriculotherapy is very efficient time-wise. Many of the students in the Auriculotherapy classes I have attended were professional acupuncturists. Their reasons for using this technology were multiple: it was quick, effective, non-invasive, the patient did not need to disrobe, needles were neither necessary to be purchased or used, puncturing the skin was not done, and infection was not an issue. In my practice, Auriculotherapy is a central practice modality.

I am aware that Auriculotherapy has a strong supporter in myself, because it is an ideal form of treatment. When paired with Ryodoraku, Auriculotherapy is unexcelled and serves primarily as a form of treatment. Ryodoraku serves more as a form of evaluation. The gentleness and non-invasiveness of both in their respective roles, with each one serving in a comfortable and effective manner, form a nearly perfect marriage of techniques.

Please be aware that there are a number of styles of Auriculotherapy, and the main two are the Chinese (thousands of years old, taken from the same medical book that classical acupuncture originated from, but is not systemized), and the French. The French system founded by Dr. Nogier in the 1950's is more detailed, modern, systemized, physically-oriented, and practical.

The French system is even capable of treating on the cellular level. I use both, but mainly the French system. Auriculotherapy training can be obtained by anyone, but care should be taken in order to determine whether professional licensing is a requirement, if they use needles or electrical probes, and if they are using the Chinese system or the French. I am an instructor in Auriculotherapy and do present seminars in this art. I teach mainly the French method, but also some of the Chinese system and I only use electrical methods, not needles.

I can be contacted at billeasleydc@yahoo.com for further information regarding Auriculotherapy training. If only an interest in the topic is what is intended, then purchasing the Manual of Auriculotherapy by Terry Oleson, Ph.D. (I prefer the 2nd. edition) would likely be your best option. An interesting thing to mention here is that a significant number of classical (needle-using) acupuncturists attend our classes due to the efficiency and effectiveness of the system.

CLASSIC ACUPUNCTURE

ANOTHER FINE ART

One of the main purposes of this book is to provide a less complex way of working with the meridian system, indeed, the entire energy system of the human being.

Acupuncture, as practiced in traditional Chinese medicine, is truly a fine art...and a complex art. It takes years of study and practice to produce even a mediocre practitioner. There are nearly 30 different pulses to master the reading, interpretation, and differentiation of plus understanding how to apply this information to the system and have a positive effect without making things worse. Acupuncture is polarizing/depolarizing in nature, while Auriculotherapy is normalizing in nature.

In my practice, I have neither the time nor the inclination to delve deeply into acupuncture because there are practical and effective alternatives. Besides the foregoing, as a Doctor of Chiropractic in my state, using needles in acupuncture was not legal plus I don't like using needles anyway. Once I learned that micro-current via an electrical probe worked just as well, I simply dispensed with the idea of needles.

Since one of the main intentions of this book is to not have to go through the arduous training required in traditional acupuncture but rather a less arduous one as presented in this offering, this section is accordingly brief.

IN CONCLUSION

Hopefully, the content of this book has brought the reader to the understanding that human beings are twice as complex as previous believed by the conventional system of health care. Many have suffered because of conventional medicine's focus on the physical aspect only.

One of the main purposes for this book is to bring to the forefront of the reader's mind that there is another entire dimension to both health and disease, and how it may be incorporated for the healing of many health issues not properly addressed in both the past and present.

Furthermore, the methods presented herein will hopefully enable many capable and devoted healers to engage in the healing arts and fill the large gap left by the conventional system of treatment without having to go through the arduous and lengthy training of traditional acupuncture. One of the intentions of those from whom I learned these methods was to provide a much more abbreviated, but even more effective, system of healing certain conditions. This is not intended to replace traditional acupuncture, but augment it for the well-being of people everywhere.

APPENDIX

SUMMARY OF DIFFERENTIATING BETWEEN ENERGY-BASED AND PHYSICALLY-BASED DISEASE

Physically-based diseases are easily and reliably diagnosed by conventional methods such as X-ray, lab tests, etc. The physical signs and symptoms caused by energy based diseases are frequently also diagnosable. The difference is that even after tests, with energy-based conditions the doctors can tell you what is happening but not why. They can offer treatments to handle the symptoms, but not full healing.

Physicians are very intelligent and observant, and base their conclusions on empirical evidence. These observations are used to develop a name or identity to a pattern of symptoms with which the entire conventional medical community then agrees – if for nothing else political and industrial management purposes. This is the partial cause of some aspects of "cookbook medicine" in which the doctor identifies a symptom pattern and calls it whatever they have been taught by others to call it, who likewise did not know what its cause was, then follow these established treatment protocols however ineffective. What other choice do they have?

What results from this is that someone goes to their doctor for some legitimate health concern; their physician refers them for testing, and often to a specialist who gives their condition a name. There the ball is dropped. With no defined standard medical protocol of treatment that results in full healing, the circus begins trying to find a way to deal with the issue, usually an ineffective albeit costly one.

Foundational aspects of history-taking are the questions: How did this happen? When did this happen? Why did this happen? Is there an infection? If so, what are the details? Is there an injury? If so, what are the details?

MOST IMPORTANT is that if these foundational questions do not have a clear and direct answer, the problem is very, very likely of energetic origin...no matter what the previous health care professional may have called it. They could very well have been correct in diagnosis, but have no plan for complete resolution of the condition. All they can offer is pain killers or other chemical concoctions with a list of negative side effects as long as your arm.

To use a typical and obvious example, that of a fractured arm:

- Has a distinct history that is very definite and recognizable (Doc, I fell off a ladder and broke my arm).

- Has pain patterns that are characteristic for their perceived origin (the fractured arm). Their arm hurts.

- Responds to conventional physically-based treatment (the placement of a cast).

- Has a predictable healing pattern (it will have a lump on it for a long time).

- Has a predictable prognosis (six weeks with a cast, then be careful for another six weeks and there will be some muscle loss).

- The pain involved follows classic neurologic patterns, anatomy, and physiology.

- No matter how many doctors are consulted, they generally agree on the treatment, diagnosis, and prognosis.

- Change of physical position or posture often does change the symptoms.

- Change of emotional status and mood does not result in a change of symptoms.

- Nearly every doctor consulted will employ identical diagnostic methods (X-ray).

• Generally speaking, the whole process will be both expected and consistent throughout.

• Biopsy can be useful in certain cases other than fracture.

For chest pain, changing physical position may help differentiate between musculoskeletal problems and cardiac problems. A change of position, pronounced breathing, or other movement, will exacerbate the musculoskeletal condition, but will not likely affect a cardiac condition.

Energetically-based are mysterious in origin. To use a typical and obvious example, that of irritable bowel syndrome (there are no laboratory, clinical, or diagnostic tests for irritable bowel syndrome, only the complaints of the sufferer):

• Has no distinct onset, clinical methods do not readily reveal any recognizable pathology (the history lacks any determining feature, such as an accident or even a precise date, which translates to, "Doc, it just sneaked up on me, and I don't know just when it started – maybe 4 or 5 years ago.").

• The pain patterns are not consistent with normal anatomy and physiology (only generalized cramps, nothing specific).

• Does not respond well to conventional treatment (only general physiology-altering medicines have any effect, which is actually treating the symptom, not the disease; therefore, it never goes away).

• Does not have a predictable healing pattern (the doctor cannot give reasonable information regarding prognosis on this beyond vague guesses).

• Attempted prognoses are useless (with no real information to go on, all the doctor can do is make vague guesses).

• Change of physical position or posture often does change the symptoms.

- Change of emotional status and mood does not result in a change in symptoms.

- No matter how many doctors are consulted, they generally agree on the treatment, and diagnosis, but don't know the cause. In this case, the symptoms are so obvious that anyone can guess as well as the doctor; but in cases such as fibromyalgia, migraines, asthma, and other "mystery" diseases, the only thing the doctors have to go on are physical symptoms with no physical abnormalities whatsoever, with the exception of functional findings, which is what the patient tells them in the first place. So, with the weird pains and problems some people have, no matter how many doctors they consult, their problem forever remains a mystery.

- Prognosis is an unknown (a lot of vague guesses populate this area of concern).

- The pain involved does not follow classic neurologic patterns, anatomy, and physiology.

- Nearly every doctor consulted will employ identical diagnostic methods if they are making the same guesses; but if they are guessing differently, they will likely order a variety of tests which often results in a different diagnosis. The problem is that they are examining the results without understanding the cause.

- Generally speaking, the whole process will be both confused and inconsistent throughout; unless of course, the doctors are making similar guesses which of late, they seem to be better at, albeit wrong guesses nonetheless.

- The more doctors consulted the more confused it gets with all the differing diagnoses.

- Treatment not only varies depending on the practitioner but does not work effectively.

- Biopsy is of no use as it comes back normal.

Don't be confused by functionally-named diseases. Examples include irritable bowel syndrome (IBS), premenstrual syndrome (PMS), carpal tunnel syndrome (CTS), fibromyalgia (which means muscle fiber pain), reflex sympathetic dystrophy (RSD) also called complex regional pain syndrome (CRPS), and others. You might notice the acronyms involved and remember that "S" stands for "syndrome", which means a collection of symptoms in which, when a certain number of these are found together, they then constitute that "disease".

Remember symptoms are the result of disease not the disease itself, nor their cause. They are naming the symptom or result, not the cause, the behavior, not the reason for that behavior - a metaphor for this is attempting to correct a child's bad behavior rather than the reason such behavior is present to begin with. A crying baby is one example. A baby always has a reason when they cry; so don't punish the baby, investigate instead. A child always has a reason behind misbehavior, and a misbehaving tissue (asthma, cramps, IBS) always has a reason based on the influences that regulate that tissue's behavior and for doing what it is or isn't doing.

It cannot be stressed strongly enough to understand why something is happening and why so many energetically-based diseases have been given "mainstream medical names". The conventional medical industry treats these misunderstood conditions endlessly, which results in endless income and political power for them to continue their endless and expensive research. This capability is derived from the ignorance the general population suffers in terms of understanding why they are not well and desiring a greater state of health on a personal basis or for a loved one.

It seems we have learned how to kill ourselves more slowly and have amortized our suicide on the installment plan to longer terms and have a lot of money change hands in the process.

It is well to remember that while the conventionally educated professional may mistake many energetically-based diseases for physically-based ones; it is also just as important to be aware that the energetically-based healer may do just the opposite – that of mistaking a physically-based disease for an energetically-based one. It is for this reason that the conventional, physically-based educational and training recommendations are set forth in the body of the text of this book.

These recommendations are not to be taken lightly. It is the convert from the traditional professions to the mystical and energetic that is the least likely to mistake a physically-based disease for an energetic one. The Easley Energy Therapy Treatment Manual, soon to be released and available separately, is simple enough for anyone with an 8th grade education to apply to heal themselves and their family members. However, if your intention is to practice with the general public, additional education is essential.

The following worksheet is included to assist the practitioner in determining whether a condition is physically based or energetic, or a combination. A physically based condition will have most of the check marks in the Yes column, and an energetically based condition in the No column. A mixed condition will be fairly evenly distributed between both.

PHYSICAL/ENERGETIC BASIS OF CONDITION

Question	Yes	No
Does the condition have a clear origin?		
Are the symptoms consistent with the origin?		
Have any medical treatments been effective long term?		
Has there been a predictable pattern of healing?		
Does the pain follow expected patterns? (i.e. nerve pathways)		
Has the progression been predictable?		
Have previous doctors consistently agreed?		
Have previous doctors used similar tests?		
Is the pain or symptoms consistent, does not change with moods?		
Do the symptoms change with physical position?		
Has the process of healing gone as expected?		
If a biopsy was performed, was it helpful?		

EXPLANATION OF TERMS

Please see below the detailed information on terms mentioned as treatment or advice in the list of conditions and their treatment:

Acupuncture: It is expected that any practitioner engaged in anything resembling acupuncture have sufficient knowledge and training in this art. It is also expected that anyone engaging in meridian work would have on hand the texts and manuals that would supply the practitioner with the appropriate information with which to perform quality work. With that having been said, the information set out in this book does not and is not intended to present identical information found in classic acupuncture. Easley Energy Therapy (EET) is a different system than acupuncture that has been recently developed, but does incorporate some of the meridian and acupuncture/reflex points found in classic acupuncture. EET is compatible with the other therapies presented in this text. It has a deep relationship with these other therapies because it was from the knowledge learned through these other systems that EET grew and came into being. The use of more than one treatment modality is a holistic and more complete system of healing.

Clinical treatment note: The treatment time per point is around eight seconds. While this may seem very brief to the classic acupuncturist, clinically, it works very, very well. This has been proven by the author in clinical application. As has been mentioned, this is a different system; and it is very efficient.

Auriculotherapy: The micro-current evaluation and treatment of ear points according to both the European (French) and Chinese systems. I do not suggest the use of needles, but I do suggest a micro-current probe utilizing equipment that registers the electrical character of the point in question. While this equipment may be quite expensive, the minimum I would advise is a unit that delivers ten cycles per second and has a "point finder". I use the Electro Medical Stim Flex 400A which is a medically registered unit.

The typical treatment time per point is eight seconds and normally no more than 16 seconds. There are, of course, exceptions to this general rule.

Also, I recommend the protocols found in either the Electro Medical Association's printed material or in the Auriculotherapy Manual. This can be used by a beginner with confidence; but when getting into the advanced levels, such as the 4 phases of the ear, taking a class is strongly recommended.

Balanced, organic, and low glycemic: These are generalities that the practitioner is not only expected to be familiar with but to be very knowledgeable in. Fads have no place in true healing. Know your food and dietary material and know it with confidence. When in doubt, consider the most natural of choices that have been around the longest.

Behavior modification: Refers to the practice of refraining from doing things that are counter to the goals of the therapy and engaging in the doing of things that promote the goals of the therapy. This could pertain to nearly any kind of changing of how things are done; and for this reason, it is advisable that the practitioner have an adequate grasp of appropriate changes that would be beneficial for the patient.

Chakras: The chakras listed are the ones that seem related, either directly or indirectly, to the problem. It is a good thing to know that simply adding energy to a problem area may prove problematic without first extracting the diseased and corrupted energies. For further information, I recommend Master Choa Kok Sui's book, 'The Chakras and Their Functions."

Coffee enema: This is an old remedy but may be strange and new to many patients. According to those who taught me the value of coffee as a healing agent, it is the color of the energy of the coffee; therefore, it is the frequency and energy of the coffee that enables it to function as it does. There may well be chemical (such as caffeine) or hormonal attributes to it as well, but what is important is that it does what it does. In this instance, the caffeine is delivered directly to the liver via the hepatic portal system and speeds up the metabolism of the liver. The rest of the body is unaffected.

Never introduce hot coffee into the lower gastrointestinal tract...ever. Allow it to cool to body temperature. The temperature is not the mechanism of treatment. In general, the purpose of the use of coffee is to cleanse the system. Specialized coffees are not necessary. It is sufficient to use the least expensive regular coffee available.

For daily enemas, large quantities are not necessary; and it is recommended to hold the coffee in the system for around 20 minutes. If more than a pint is introduced to the body, it is less likely the individual will be comfortable retaining it very long. If this becomes problematic, several short duration enemas can be done instead.

Coffee energetically cleanses the basic and sex chakras and the associated meridians and nadis. It is also very effective at cleaning the colon when used in greater amounts, up to two liters; and with the colon in a higher state of cleanliness, the liver is also detoxified. When engaging in these in-depth cleanses, progressive amounts of water are introduced until the colon is completely devoid of fecal matter and the water comes out clear. The coffee is used as the second last enema, and the last is clear water. It should be noted that the colon has as a primary function, withdrawing the liquid from the feces in order to enable a proper bowel movement; and this withdrawn liquid is moved into the bloodstream and transported directly to the liver for processing and detoxifying via the hepatic portal vein.

Small daily enemas are fine and a good idea, but very thorough colonics should be limited to once a week at the most unless there is a very good reason to do so. Violation of this principle may result in disruption of the bowel flora population.

Colonic: A professionally rendered colonic irrigation that is intended to cleanse the entire large intestine but not including the addition of other substances or gases.

Earthing: Earthing is the practice of re-establishing your electrical connection with beloved Mother Earth. It is one of the most powerful of antioxidants. Some people are aware that attaching a grounding strap to an automobile will help prevent the formation of rust which is oxidation. Earthing is essentially the same thing, but it has the effect of neutralizing the inappropriate electrical charges in the body. This is done by going barefoot, particularly effective when walking in grass wet with dew in the morning. It lowers the viscosity of the blood, lowers blood pressure, relieves inflammation, and slows the aging process; plus, it's very inexpensive.

Lifestyle changes and recommendations: This is a reference to actually changing one's lifestyle and habits in a positive and meaningful way. If this means massive change, so be it. Sometimes it's easier to develop a whole new, healthier lifestyle than change the old, unhealthy, self-destructive one, one painful part at a time. A good healthy proper diet, exercise, and mental habit improvements are expected as a general rule. Positive thinking, non-judgment, and always trying to do the right thing are also expected. If a patient wants their life to remain miserable, avoiding these foundational changes will guarantee it.

Ideally, half of one's lifestyle is physical and the other half is spiritual. To help explain it, we are dual in nature. We are human beings, meaning "human" and "being"...half physical and half spiritual. Positive thought and non-reaction are part of spirituality. One does not have to meditate and pray half of the time in order to be spiritual. It's more a lifestyle than an isolated practice.

Meditation: This refers to the most balanced set of meditations that people can use without generating problems for themselves. I use Grand Master Choa Kok Sui's Meditation on Twin Hearts as a primary basis for a healing meditation. It is available in three forms: one is the general meditation; the other two contain additions at the end specifically for the purpose of enabling physical healing or psychological healing. A fourth meditation very useful for general development and balance is the Meditation on the Lord's Prayer (also from Grand Master Choa Kok Sui). All of these meditations have a gentle exercise included that is to be done before and after the meditation proper. Generally speaking, I do not use simple, silent, relaxing types of meditation; because the same amount of time can be applied to greater benefit with the ones just recommended. More information on this can be found at www.pranichealing.com

Miasm: From classical homeopathy, "The term miasm can be defined most easily as "pollution"; a base pollution to a living organism giving rise to chronic as well as some acute illness." When the term "miasm" is used in this book, it refers to a pathological influence to the spiritual components, such as nadis, or other foundational energetic structure that persists from one incarnation to the next, incarnation after incarnation. In this fashion, a "miasm" is 'inherited' from an earlier incarnation via the timeless component of a major nadi, or possibly from a genetic source, such as one's parent or grandparent, or other ancestor. Imagine it as spiritual pollution that affects the performance of one's genetic, or non-genetically dictated functioning.

Organic, natural diet: The consumption of foods, preferably home-grown, organic, of a wide variety, and hopefully used according to one's blood type.

Pranic Healing: This is a complete set of skills and knowledge. It is detailed, and the texts involved contain protocols for many, many conditions. For the practitioner, it is expected that he or she have these texts physically on hand and refer to them every time a protocol is being used. I feel it should be stated here that we are doing healing not playing at healing. This is serious business. Pranic Healing shares a relatively close relationship with Reiki, and many Pranic Healing practitioners are also Reiki masters.

There is truly a hierarchy in the spiritual worlds, and the healer's function is to plug connect with that structure in a proper and effective manner as a conduit for the healing energies. The healer then conveys these blessings to the patient, the true recipient. It's not about the importance of the healer but about delivering the blessings and healing energies by the method most efficient for accomplishing that task.

Pranic Healing can be done at a distance. Please keep in mind that the more open the connection is between the healer and the patient, the greater the likelihood for the success of the session.

The website for Pranic Healing in the United States is www.pranichealing.com

Probiotics: This is a general reference to the practice of the ingestion of a supplemental gut flora microbial population. There are many of these on the market. It also refers to the ingestion of fermented foods which are actually more complete and less expensive. These cultures are commercially available. Typically, fermented foods contain about 1,000 times the number of beneficial microbes compared to the commercially available supplements found in bottles. The importance of this therapy cannot be understated, particularly in instances where psychological and mental/mood function is an issue. This is quickly becoming more widely used as the health care community is beginning to understand its importance.

Ryodoraku: This is a system of evaluation and treatment of the acupuncture meridian system. It is the electronic version of pulse reading and gives the practitioner an electrical conductance/resistance value from zero to 200 on each point. These readings are then compared to one another to determine the course of treatment and also what not to treat. In very complicated cases, where there are so many positive readings that only further confusion would result from a normal treatment, treat both left and right Spleen 21 points on the side of the rib cage and have the patient come back for another treatment on another day. The equipment I use is the Electro Meridian Imaging (EMI) instrument which is associated with the International Academy of Medical Acupuncture. This organization is one of the best and has been around a long time. They are also suppliers of quality supplies. Their website is www.iama.edu

Supplementation: This refers to using nutritional supplements that you know work, and my inclusions here are what I know about it. I am not a professional clinical nutritionist, so do your research, use your knowledge, as these are only basic suggestions.

Treatment modalities and protocols: This refers to a general, but flexible set of practices and philosophies in which the practitioner is proficient. The intent of this book is to offer an expansion of these skills and knowledge or the opportunity to acquire additional skills and knowledge.

What this means is use what you know; as there are many comparable treatment modalities, each dependant on practitioner skill and compatibility.

Salt water bath: This refers to the age-old practice of using salt as a spiritual cleansing agent. The quality of salt is not important, so obtain the least expensive available. Rock salt is too lumpy for bathing, so use granulated salt. Bathing in ocean water is ideal if available. The way this functions is that the salt breaks up and disintegrates the energies, and the water holds these energies so they can be disposed of.

Note: this practice removes all forms of energy equally; so, therefore, lounging around in a salt bath can be exhausting. Limit time in a salt bath to 20 minutes. A salt shower can be also done. To do this, simply wet the body; step away from or divert the shower stream; sprinkle salt over the entire body, and rub gently and make sure to treat all the less exposed parts, such as arm pits, etc.; as they serve as pockets for stagnant energy. Wait 2 -3 minutes for the salt to do its work. After this simply rinse the salt off with water. This is to be done after the soap phase of showering.

Yogic alternate nostril breathing or simply yogic breathing: This is a commonly known practice of breathing in through one nostril, usually beginning with the left, and out the right nostril, then breathing in the right nostril, and out the left. There is a cadence to this of counting a certain number of seconds in some styles of alternate breathing. It begins after an initial exhalation, then inhale through the left nostril to a count of 6 seconds, then hold for one second, then exhale through the right nostril for a count of 6 seconds. Hold the breath out for a count of one second, and then inhale through the right nostril for a count of 6 seconds, hold for one second, and exhale through the left nostril for a count of 6 seconds. This is one cycle. This should be done for 7 cycles.

In brief it goes: in left for 6, hold one, out right for 6, hold one, in right for 6, hold for one, out left for 6, hold for one. The concept is whichever nostril you breathe out of, you inhale through that nostril; and whichever nostril you breathe in to, you breathe out of the other one. Do not violate the recommendation of doing only 7 cycles. This is very powerful; and when done improperly or in excess, it can throw one's system out of balance.

REFERENCED MATERIALS AND RECOMMENDED READING LIST

The following is a list of books referred to in this book and a partial list of highly recommended additional reading:

Dorland's Medical Dictionary
The Prophet by Kahlil Gibran
Touch For Health by John F. Thie (Applied Kinesiology)
Hole's Human Anatomy and Physiology textbook
Contact Reflex Analysis – An Energy Connection
        by Dr. Dick A. Versendaal
The Unseen Self, Revised: Kirlian Photography Explained
        by Brian Snellgrove
The Five Elements of Self-Healing: Using Chinese Medicine for Maximum Immunity, Wellness, and Health
        by Jason Elias and Katherine Ketcham
Various books and programs by Tony Robbins
The German New Medicine by Dr. Ryke Geerd Hamer
MMS HEALTH RECOVERY GUIDEBOOK 1st Edition
        by Jim Humble
The Cancer Cure That Worked: 50 Years of Suppression
        by Barry Lynes
Thought Forms by Annie Besant and C.W. Leadbeater
The Chakras by C.W. Leadbeater
Ryodoraku acupuncture: A guide for the application of Ryodoraku therapy : electrical acupuncture, a new autonomic nerve regulating therapy
        by Yoshio Nakatani
Manual of Auriculotherapy by Terry Oleson, PhD.

Books by Master Choa Kok Sui:
Miracles Through Pranic Healing, Pranic Psychotherapy, Advanced Pranic Healing, The Chakras and Their Functions, and The Spiritual Essence of Man

Bible references from the New American Standard Bible, Published by Holman Bible Publishers

ABOUT THE AUTHOR

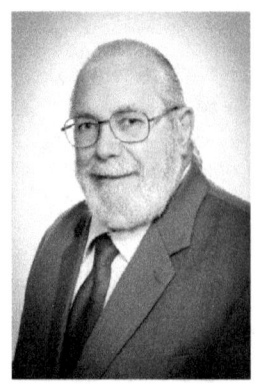

Dr. Easley's extensive qualifications include:

Doctorate in Chiropractic
Doctorate in Alternative Healing
Certified practitioner of Auriculotherapy
Post-doctoral faculty in Auriculotherapy
Professor of Human Anatomy & Physiology, university level
Live Blood Microscopy (phase contrast & dark field)
Acupuncture
Certified in Meridian Energetics and Ryodoraku
Pranic Healing Basic, Advanced, Post Advanced, Psychotherapy, Crystal, and Psychic Self Defense levels
Applied Kinesiology
Reiki, and many other qualifications

Numerous qualifications in traditional medical areas (diagnostics, radiology, physical therapy, pain management, etc.)

Ordained minister (actual ordination, not mail order)

Founder and developer of Easley Energy Therapy, the system of treatment presented in this volume.

Dr. Easley lives in Cuenca, Ecuador.

www.ingramcontent.com/pod-product-compliance
Lightning Source LLC
Chambersburg PA
CBHW052312220526
45472CB00001B/82